Mad[illegible] Scotland

D O Gregory

chipmunkapublishing
the mental health publisher

Published by
Chipmunkapublishing
United Kingdom

http://www.chipmunkapublishing.com

ISBN 978-1-84991-986-9

Chipmunkapublishing gratefully acknowledge the support of Arts Council England.

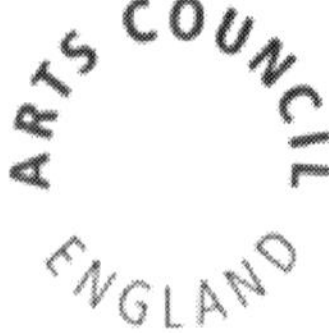

CONTENTS

INTRODUCTION

Made in Scotland is the Biography of a Refugee in the UK who was diagnosed in 2008 with Paranoid Schizophrenia, who is now living in Scotland from an African descent. This book talks about the place, time and country of birth of Simon Oghenejiro Algood.; his family background and growing up as a child. It talks about his primary, secondary and University education and the history of his mental illness, how it started and his relocation to the UK.

In this book you will find out more about Schizophrenia, its signs, symptoms and causes. As you read on this book describes the author's stages in life as a mental health patient and relationship breakdown. It shows the essence of being in a family and a healthy relationship. It talks about the most difficult part of the author's life. He has taken time to write this book and this is the best way he could explain in detail the difficulties in his life and how he overcame them in the end. The author has used a pseudonym for every name in this book to protect the privacy of the individuals and also the locations have been changed.

Made in Scotland is a book the author would recommend to everyone especially those with mental health issues, refugees or asylum seekers and mental health professionals. It's a book that will help you build confidence, be independent and teach you how to stay strong and to be in the right relationship and believe in GOD almighty. This is a true life story which the author is confidently telling you with honesty. This is a book that will inspire you to become what you want to become and achieve your goal.

I hope as you read you will be drawn to the right decision in your life and overcome every obstacle just as the author did in the end. Enjoy your reading.

CHAPTER ONE
GROWING UP AND FAMILY HISTORY
THE BIOGRAPHY OF SIMON OGHENEJIRO ALGOOD

Simon Oghenejiro Algood was born into the family of Wisdom Algood and Beatrice Rosemary Akpan in Ebutte Metta in Lagos State of Nigeria on the 20th March 1979. His mother was a citizen of the Federal Republic of Nigeria from Etinan Local Government area of Akwa Ibom State and his father was a citizen of the Federal Republic of Nigeria from Algood Quarters, Otujeremi Town, Ughelli South Local Government Area of Delta State.

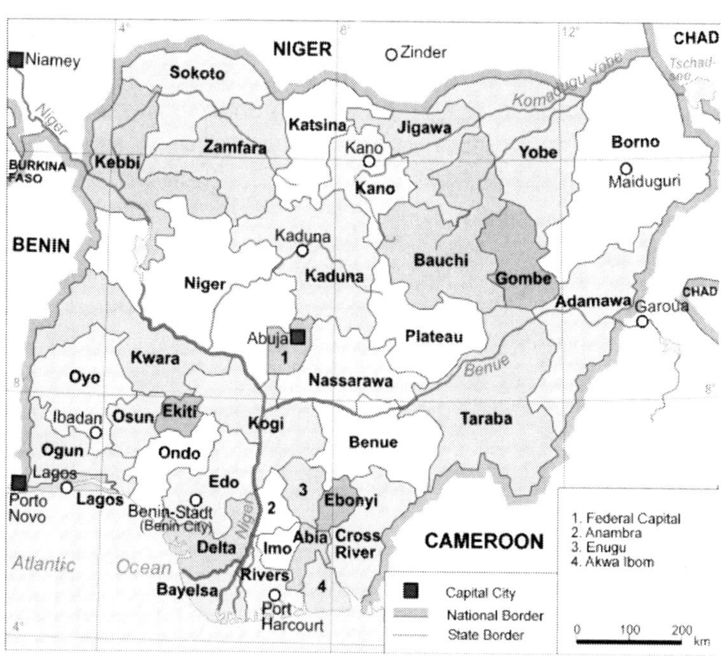

Simon's country of birth, Nigeria is a federal constitutional republic which comprises 36 states and its Federal Capital Territory, Abuja. Nigeria is located in West Africa and shares land borders with the Republic of Benin in the west, Chad and Cameroon in the east, and Niger Republic in the north. Its coast in the south lies on the Gulf of Guinea on the Atlantic Ocean. The three largest and most influential ethnic groups in Nigeria are the Hausa, Igbo and Yoruba. There are other recognized regional languages like Edo, Efik, Ibibio, Kanuri, Fulani, Idoma, Ijaw, Urhobo, Ilaje, Isoko, Itsekiri , Ebira, Nupe, Gwari, Jukun, Igala, Tiv and others. Pidgin English is another widely spoken language outside the English language, it is spoken throughout Nigeria and it is also known as "Broken" (Broken English).

Nigeria has more than 250 ethnic groups, with varying languages and customs, creating a country of rich ethnic diversity. The number of languages currently estimated and catalogued in Nigeria is 521. This number includes 510 living languages, two second languages without native speakers and nine extinct languages. In some areas of Nigeria, ethnic groups speak more than one language. The official language of Nigeria, English, was chosen to facilitate the cultural and linguistic unity of the country. The choice of English as the official language was partially related to the fact that a part of the Nigerian population spoke English as a result of British Colonization that ended in 1960.

Nigeria is the most populous country in Africa, the seventh most populous country in the world, and the most populous country in the world in which the majority of the population is black. The present day Nigeria has a population of just over 150 million people. The people of Nigeria have an extensive history. Archaeological evidence had shown that human habitation of the area dates back to at least 9000 BC. The area around the

Benue and Cross River is thought to be the original homeland of the Bantu migrants who spread across most of central and southern Africa in waves between the 1st millennium BC and the 2nd millennium. Nigeria is roughly split between Muslims in the North and Christians in the South; a very small minority practice traditional religion or who are called animist.

Simon grew up to know that Jesus Christ was the saviour of the World and he died to redeem us of our sins through his Mother Beatrice. Simon's mother was born into a Christian family of the catholic faith. All members of his mother's family are baptised and bear their baptismal name. Simon's mother was a trader selling groceries while his father worked with Nigeria Tobacco Company and he retired at a point and was working as a driver delivering goods for customers at a particular time.

Simon's parents never had a perfect relationship, they were always quarrelling and sometimes his father beat up his mother. Simon's father was a heavy smoker and he was also a heavy drinker. All the care he ever had came from his mother although his father sometimes contributed whenever he was in his right senses.

As a child Simon and his family lived in different places in Lagos. He could remember they lived in Ebutte-Metta where he was born, Baddia, Alaba, Ojo Road, Okokomaiko, Agric (along badagry expressway), Ajangbadi and in Abgara Estate in Ogun State. There are other places his parents lived in Lagos before he was born but he didn't mention them in this book. Lagos is one of the most populated cities in Nigeria. When Simon was growing up, Christmas was always a special day and it's the only time they ate chicken. Coming from a very poor background, certain things they see or observe which are supposed to be a normal way of life but are seen as affluence in the society. In those days owning a car, a house, a coloured TV, a video cassette recorder or having an air conditioner at home were not seen as a necessity by a majority of the population.

Christmas is also the time when everyone wore their best clothes, shoes and shocks bought by their parents. They always wear different clothes for Christmas and New Year. It's traditional in those days to always wear new clothes over this festive period. During this period there are often fireworks lit up in the sky especially on New Year's Eve where no one sleeps throughout the night. Fireworks are generally known as "banga and bisco" in the common pidgin dialect. 31st December is often called "watch night of new year". Festive seasons like Christmas, New Year, Easter etc. are well marked and recognised among Christians in Nigeria, even those who don't go to Church throughout the year never miss Church on New Year's eve. New Year's Eve is a time when people make resolution to GOD especially, and to their loved ones and about their life if they need a change or turnaround. This period is also a time when people visit friends, neighbours or relatives. The festive period always brings joy among people and everyone enjoys the public holiday as well. There are always lots to eat this period. Those who don't have much to eat or no food at all will always visit others with the aim of having something to eat after staying for some hours. Sometimes they are often given money as a Christmas present instead of food. Nigeria use to be a nice place to live at that time, it's so different now from the present day Nigeria.

Simon had never wanted to live in Nigeria even from his childhood. Simon could remember when he was about seven years old before he started primary school, his mother bought him a safe, and it was known as "colo" in the local dialect. He would put any money he had in there from time to time and would tell his family members that he is saving money to travel overseas when he grows up. They would laugh at him and say "do you know how long it will take you to save up till you re grown up before you will travel"? Don't you think as you become older you will use the money for other things? He would say no he won't use it for other things; He has only ever wanted to travel overseas and be there all his life. His favourite place in the World has been the UK right from his childhood. He always kept his safe in a hidden place.

If anyone needed money at that time he always offered to be a lender but would demand interest in return. This made one of his elder sister's Patricia gave him the nickname "Shylock". She also gave him the nickname "Old Man" because he looked much smaller and younger than his age. There are other nicknames he was known as by his family members and which are very popular among his extended family which he has not mentioned in this book.

In those days every member of his family had nicknames and it was fun to have nicknames. Sometimes people around like calling you by your nickname even when they know your name. Although it depends on the kind of nicknames, it often leads to quarrels and a fight when you are been coined a new nickname which you might not like. Sometimes parents call their children by their nicknames given to them by their friends at school which makes everything even more fun.

Growing up as a child was quite fun not until Simon was about eleven years old. Although before this time there were always ups and downs in his family but he never ever felt the impact that much until he was eleven.
Simon's mother taught the children to pray, the Lord's Prayer and bed time poem, most of them he can't remember apart from a few lines from the poem "My

Mother". Sometimes at night before bed time, his mother always gathered the children and talked to them about GOD and taught them about manners. She always told them how they used to behave when they were babies and they picked up nicknames for each other from stories being told by their mother. Simon's mother was like everything to all of the children at that time even though his father was present in the house.

He was the fifth child in his family of seven children. The First was Charlie, the second Patricia, then Ruth, Henry, Simon, Hannah and Jason. Charlie is a very tall and handsome man, dark, quiet, hardworking, focused and easy going. Paricia is a beautiful woman, tall, with pointed nose, very light skinned like their mother and looks very much like her. Ruth is known as the small lady in the family with pointed nose, bright eyes and brilliant. Henry, his immediate elder brother is the most brilliant among the family; he is light skinned, average in height and highly skilled and very smart. Simon is very quiet, average in height, brown skin, brown eyes, black hair, and funny sometimes, good build even though he looked small in his childhood, organised and very reserved. Hannah his immediate younger sister is just about the same height as him, brilliant, brown skin, black hair and a nice person. Jason is average in height, hardworking, brown skin and a very nice person as well.
Simon's family is a very large one as you can see and when he was growing up there was love between each one of them. They respected their parents though they never learnt how to speak their parent's local dialect because they were brought up in the Pidgin language they only learnt English language from school.

CHAPTER TWO
SIMON'S EDUCATION AND FAMILY BREAKDOWN

Simon started Primary school in January 1987; the name of his Primary school was L.A. Primary School at Alaba Oro in Lagos State. He was 8 years old by then. He should have started school earlier but because he had a diminutive stature, whenever his mother took him to register for school he was always turned back by the registrars because they didn't believe his age. He was lucky to be accepted for school that year. In those days they allow you to put your right hand on the top of your head and tell you to allow your middle finger to reach the bottom of your left ear, if it doesn't touch or reach the bottom of the ear then it means you're too young to start school. That was the system they used in those days in Nigeria to admit people into school.

Simon was an average student during his primary school education, his family members always saw him as being dull when it came to academics. There was a time he came home with position 13th of a class of about 28. At this time everyone in his family were saying different things about him and were not happy with his result. However, his elder brother Henry looked at his result and called the attention of the family members and explained that he did well because his percentage was around 70, which meant there were brilliant pupils in the class at that time. This made them consider changing their minds and stop calling him names. Simon's younger sister was much more brilliant than him when they were growing up because she had the opportunity to go to a nursery school for three years before she started primary school. Simon struggled through his primary school but was able to go through and finish the six years.

Simon finished his Primary school in June 1992 and proceeded to continue his secondary education at Odofin Secondary School, Mile 2, Lagos State. He was the clown of his class and everyone liked him. He enjoyed his secondary school days. There he came to meet other pupils who came from different primary schools and were admitted to the same secondary school as himself. During this time there was fierce competition in terms of academic abilities of individuals. Simon began to pick up in his academic ability and this was when he would say he became brilliant and was one of the big names in his class.

He sat for his Junior Secondary Certificate Examination in 1995 and passed all his subjects and went on to Senior Secondary Education where he sat for his Senior Secondary Certificate Examination in June 1998. At this time he did not pass English Language and Physics. His school's performance that year was very poor; only four students at the time passed English Language. He enrolled again for the Examination in 1999 at Federal Government Secondary School and he passed all his subjects in just one sitting including English Language and Physics. He also enrolled for G.C.E. examinations in 1999 and passed all his subjects in one sitting. G.C.E. examinations are often taken in November/December each year for those who didn't make up their subjects in the S.S.C.E in May/Jun. G.C.E and W.A.S.S.C.E. are examinations recognised in West Africa. At present there are other examination body that award certificates that are recognised in Nigeria. During this time he changed his first name to his middle name. So he was known as Simon Oghenejiro Algood. In Nigeria, they always write the surname first, followed by the first name and then the middle name. So when he was in Nigeria his name was always written as Algood Simon Oghenejiro. Simon worked as a Sales Man in a cement shop briefly for a few months after his secondary school education and was able to gather some money. He also worked as a factory worker in a plastic company for over a year before he got admission to the University.

Simon almost stopped school at a point in time because his father refused to send him to school. His father had seven children from his mother and he was not responsible towards any of the children. There was a rich man call Mr Peter Oghenejiro Orevaoghene who was one of Simon's neighbours, he took responsibility for his education when he was in the fourth year of his secondary education up till the end of his University education. Mr Orevaoghene was his name sake because they both share the same middle name.

There was a time when he was in his secondary school that his father was really treating them so bad, this was some years after he separated with his mother at this time he almost stopped school because of the pressure. Any time they do wrong him, he would drive them out of the house telling them to take their belongings and leave to go anywhere. Most times it took the intervention of neighbours to make him change his mind. This attitude by his father led to disperse and division in the family. Simon's father never knew how to love his family. His father left them in 1991 to live with another woman who had got kids. At this time they were left with their mother, his three brothers and three sisters. At this time his mother was taking care of them selling processed corn meal, it is called "OGI" in the local dialect. His mother got money from her pastor to start up the business. They lived happily during this time and got so close to their mother.

After some years his father came with his family to beg his mother to forgive him and be allowed to come back home. His mother agreed because she has a very soft hearted woman and she was a devoted Christian. After some time living with them, his father started making trouble again. He would beat his mother up and assault her sometimes. He terrifies even his children. Sometimes when they go to school they hope that their school hours were long, they would not want to come back home because of their father. Whenever his father goes to work they would pray he did not come home on time because of what they faced. There was a time they reported their father to the police, but the police took no action saying it's a domestic issue so they can't get involved. In fact they scolded them and said how children could report their parents to the police and said we are not overseas and the culture here is different. They wanted to beat them up in the process. They asked to see his father and discussed with him then they all went home.

At this time his father became more hardened and brutal when dealing with them, most of the time he would make references about them going to the police and told them "do you think the police will be in support of a child reporting their parents"? At that time it is seen against the culture to ever go to report your parents. Whatever they tell you to do is what you do without questions. Parents are permitted to beat up their children with a whip, stick, belt or anything they want to use at that time because the society sees it as a way of disciplining the children. Sometimes they punch, slap or say abusive words to their children. They are even permitted to give very hard punishment. As a child Simon and his other brothers and sisters have gone through so many punishments. Sometimes when they wrong their parents they allow you to go to bed without saying anything to you and when you are fast asleep they wake you up with a whip and remind you of the wrong you did earlier. It could be days back but you will still serve that punishment. There were no law protecting children from parents at this time. They always seek refuge in the hands of neighbours as the case may be for days and returning home with their neighbours to plead with their parents. Sometimes when they do wrong they disappeared from home for a few hours and return home to beg their parents themselves if the neighbours are tired of pleading with their parents all the time.

Simon's father In the long run left them for the second time and they were at peace again. When the rent contract was running out his mother had no money to pay for rent and the landlady gave them quit notice. That was how his family were split again; his mother went to live with her elder sister while the rest of them went to live with their father who was living with his friend. This was in 1993. After some months he got an apartment in Ogun State where they were the caretaker. This was where he met his sponsor who helped him through his education.

Where they were living in Ogun State, was very far from his school. Simon and his younger sister had to wake up every morning at 5am to prepare to go to school. While they were living with their father, his mother always come every week to give them money for bus fare to school. Sometimes when she didn't come then they wouldn't go to school. One morning when they were preparing to go to school, He asked his father if he could assist them with money to go to school and they would pay him back when his mother comes to visit them at the weekend. He told them he had no money but said he will see what he can do. That was a lucky day for them because at least he had concern about them going to school that day. He went out and spoke to one of their neighbours who lived close by and asked if he could give his kids a lift to school.

He agreed and that was how he met his sponsor Mr Peter Oghenejiro Orevaoghene. The next day Simon and his sister went to stand in front of Mr Orevaoghene's gate, because he normally leaves at 7am. When he was about to leave they waved at him and he stopped and asked them to get in. Mr Orevaoghene told them that he could only take one person in his car because he use to pick up some other co-workers who work with him in his office along the way so the car will be filled and no room for an extra space. So the next day Simon was the only person Mr Orevaoghene picked up and his younger sister went with the public transport, but fortunately for her she got a free ride to school at a point in time from a church member. At this time after school they would walk sometimes almost 8miles to go and see their mother where she sells her groceries and get money for transport back home. They told her of the help they were getting and that made her really happy. This meant she would only be giving them money for transport back home every week instead of to and fro.

During this period his father did not change he was still living his wicked lifestyle. Anytime his mother came to visit them he tried to prevent her from seeing them and warned her not to come and visit them. There was a story that his mother told them that in their early years of courtship their father made her naked and poured fuel on her and wanted to burn her up but neighbours around intervened.

One morning they had no money for fare back home and they could not do the walking to go and see their mother after school so they decided to stay at home instead. That day was a Friday he could remember vividly well. The next day Mr Orevaoghene saw him and asked him why he didn't see him come to have a ride to school. Simon told him that his father said he had no money to give to them for transport back home and usually his mother used to support them with transport fare back home. She will be coming for the weekend as they are expecting her. The money she gave them for the week ran out so therefore that's why they stayed at home the previous day. Mr Orevaoghene said alright and said to him "do you have time later in the evening, at 5pm I want to speak with you"? He said I am free and he said meet me at home at that time.

Simon was very happy and he told his father and every member of his family that Mr Orevaoghene wants to talk with him. Everyone was anxious and wants to know what the rich man will tell him. At 5pm he rang the bell to his apartment and his domestic worker Elijah Ekong opened the door and ushered him in. He told him to have a seat while he goes upstairs to let Mr Orevaoghene know that Simon is around.

Mr Orevaoghene runs a software company and he is blessed with two kids and a beautiful wife Maria.
In few minutes he came downstairs to join him and offered him a soft drink. He began first by asking him what part of Nigeria his parents are from. He asked him if Simon was a Christian and ask him what been a Christian is to him. He then asked me how much the transport fare from his school back to home. Simon told him it is twenty naira from Mile 2 to Agbara daily and hundred naira every week. He said he should not worry he will start giving him the money for his fare back home from the next week. That was how he became his sponsor until his University. He then asked him if he will be willing to attend church with him the next day and he said sure. He told him when he normally leaves home on Sundays for church and he can come into his house at that time. Mr Orevaoghene was a very kind man. The meeting between Simon and Mr Orevaoghene didn't take more than 10 minutes and he said to him "I will see you tomorrow morning". Simon went back home very happy and told the good news to his family members, everyone was very pleased with Mr Orevaoghene and

happy for him. That was how he became a friend to Mr Orevaoghene and started attending church every Sunday with him. He attended Baptist Church with Mr Orevaoghene and his family and came to know other Christians.

At one time Mr Orevaoghene left Agbara Estate and moved to the Island of Lagos close to his work. At that time Simon didn't have time to get more contact with him but he tried to stay in touch from time to time. He joined his younger sister in following another church member to school every day. Sometimes they join their uncle, Shadrach to school because he works with one of the companies in the industrial area and drives their buses through their school to pick up workers.

Simon wrote the Joint Admissions and Matriculation Board Examination (JAMB) in 2000, this is the examination body for University admission in Nigeria and it's the equivalent of A-Level. That year candidates performed very poorly in the examination and this made Universities in Nigeria to lower the admission cut off point for different courses. He scored 221 out of 400 and he was admitted into his second choice course. The cut off point for his course that year for the University he got admission to was 200. His first choice had been Medicine but he did not make the cut off point which was 260. So he got admission in year 2000 to study for his first degree.

CHAPTER THREE
MY MENTAL HEALTH HISTORY

During Simon's studies in the University he developed some symptoms of Paranoid Schizophrenia but he was never diagnosed. Sometimes he would hear voices and hallucinate and feel he had some form of super powers. But at this time he was still able to continue his studies as this did not lead him to any hospital admission.

Simon's elder brother Charlie died in 2003 after years of suffering with Paranoid Schizophrenia. In Nigeria treatment is very poor and the proportion of budget that goes into mental health is very small or nothing at all. His brother was taken to several places for treatment including churches for prayers and traditional healing home since the medication was very scarce and expensive.

At a point in time his father gave up on him and left everything to his mother's care. Simon's mother was made a pauper just because of his brother's illness. She spent money every week running into thousands of Naira to make sure that he got well. Sometimes he saw his mother crying and he hoped that she got well and he would comfort her. His mother was the pillar of his upbringing and she always visited him at his hostel at least three times a month when he was in the University. During his time in the University he experienced withdrawal symptoms and because of his illness he heard persecutory voices and he often suspected people. As a result he started making trouble with some of his roommates. Sometimes he would not talk to them for a long period of time and if they tried to get close to him to find out what the matter was he would ignore them. At this time he became very difficult to talk to or associate with; he was just in his own World of Paranoia at that time.

Simon had a fight with one of his roommates when they were in their final year and they never talked to each other until they graduated but they are very good friends now and they take each other like brothers.

Simon graduated in 2005. He went to live with his elder sister briefly before going back to the hostel again. He went for his National Youth Service Corps (NYSC) in February 2006. NYSC means National Youth Service Corps and it is a national compulsory service for graduates who are less than 30 years of age to complete a year serving the nation. During his service he worked as a lecturer in a School of Health Technology. He made friends during his NYSC days but he has now lost contact with everyone. Simon's students liked him so much and some of them visited him at the NYSC quarters and he was the favourite among the staff in the school.

Simon finished his NYSC service on 31st January 2007. Before this time he wanted to get temporary work at the school of health but it didn't materialise, so he moved down West of Nigeria to Lagos where he grew up. He lived with a friend in Lagos. Who lived with his parents, but his parent's worked in Asaba the capital of Delta State in the South-western part of Nigeria; they do come once in a while to Lagos.

After he graduated because he could find no job and the situation in Nigeria at that time, he resorted to writing W.A.S.S.C. examinations for candidates and getting paid for it. He used the money to support his mother who started falling very ill sometimes. A friend he knew introduced him to it. He has been writing examinations for candidates before this time through his friend who

runs this illegal business. In Nigeria candidates often get leaked answers to examinations in exchange for money. He was an impersonating candidate most of the time because he got called up several times and he would negotiate the price and he would take to writing examinations for candidates. He always worked for an agent then who was his friend. He couldn't have a candidate on his own because he didn't know very well on how to go about it. He only went through an agent. Also agents always have securities put in place to protect their client. Most principals of schools take part in this business and sometimes help as security to protect the clients because they work closely with the agents and get paid for it. Most times when officials from the governing body comes to inspect schools they often give them bribes so they could allow examination malpractice to go ahead. As a client they are often given the assurance that they can't be caught by the police and they work closely with the police to keep them at bay.
Meanwhile Simon's relationship with Mr Orevaoghene had broken down earlier because, there was a time he went to him and told him that he was in a ring of people who were involved in examination malpractice and he should lend him money instead to start up a business because he didn't want to continue writing exams for people. He said he would be paying him back in instalments. This made him angry and he told Simon to leave his office. He told him that he will not stop helping him in completing his studies. From that time he lost trust with him. There was nothing else he could do to help his mother at that time or his younger siblings.

Before he moved down to Lagos, his friend has already told him that the landlady of the house had served them with a quit notice, so his coming to live with him will only be temporal. He couldn't live with his elder sister at that time because his family was divided and they were not on good terms. There was no family member he could live with not even his father at that time.

At this time his mother was a hawker. She hawked bread in the streets of Lagos. She was doing this for over 14 years and using the money he realised to take care of his sick elder brother and the other siblings. She was also homeless for more than 15 years and sleeping in a bakery all that time.

When he got to Lagos in February 2007, his aim was to leave Nigeria to find a better future for himself and to help his mother and younger siblings. Meanwhile before this time there was an addition to his family, his younger Sister Hannah had a baby girl on 30th December, 2006 and she was named Sarah.

When he was living with his friend in Lagos, Nigeria was a destabilized country. The government was full of corruption and the numbers of poor people were increasing at a very high rate. During this time, His mental state was not stable sometimes he perceived symptoms of Schizophrenia. However since he was never diagnosed he felt it was just hardship and he just needed to pray and things will get better.

There was a job interview he had at this time as a Sales Assistant in a company owned by a Lebanese. The job was for thirteen thousand naira a month (N13, 000). That's about fifty pounds and ninety eight pence (£50.98p) per month working from Monday to Friday between 8am and 5pm (9 hrs.) a day. But he turned it down because he couldn't do that kind of job as a graduate. That wage can't take him anywhere.

There was a man name Pius Dimka, he was his former neighbour when he was growing up some years back. He decided to go and meet him to see if he could help him get into the UK. He went to meet him in March 2007 to see if he could assist him to get to the UK. At first he refused, giving reasons that he might be a scammer. But he gave him his phone number to always keep in touch with him.

Simon tried to keep in touch with him at that time and at the same time he was job hunting to raise money to leave Nigeria. He went to visit him one particular day and he gave him an address and a note to give to the owner of a private Hospital in Lagos to see if he could work there for the mean time. During this time Mr Dimka was still reluctant to offer any help to him.

At a point he offered to help him to get to the UK but he gave him a condition. He said if he can help him in his office running some errands and doing any simple jobs when required. He agreed to help him. He told his mother about Mr Dimka and how he has finally agreed to help him to get to the UK and they both agree that they should go and thank him. They called him and told him they will be coming to visit him and he agreed to welcome them.

On the day they got there he called Simon privately to his office, because he uses one of the rooms in his home as his office and was questioning him. He was very angry with him and was speaking with a loud voice. He asked him why did he bring his mother to his house and he doesn't want to help him before now he has reasons not to. He warned Simon that he should never give or show anyone his statement of account. When applying for a visa you will need to submit a statement of account. Since he was supposed to act as Simon's sponsor he needed his statement of account to apply for a visa to the UK.

He was not happy with Simon and he ordered him to leave his house immediately. He handed his statement of account to him. When Simon and his mother left his house, he told his mother what he told him and she was very angry. She said she will never come to visit him any longer.

Simon went to the UK visa application centre in April 2007 but he was told by one of the members of staff that it was too early to apply for a visa since he wanted to go and study and his studies start in September. He advised him to wait till May 2007, by that time they would have started the fingerprint and eye scan introduced in the visa application.

On his way to apply for the visa, Simon was stopped by two men in clothing and they just flashed him an ID card and said there were police officers and asked to see what was in the file he was carrying. There had been some random searches going on in Lagos because of suspected crimes. He gave them the file and they saw everything and decided to arrest him saying that the documents were fake and they need to see the owner of the account. He called Mr Dimka who picked up the call and when he heard his voice he dropped it. He called him the second time but someone else picked up the call and when he asked to speak with Mr Dimka, he simply told him that Mr Dimka has travelled. He started sensing something was really going wrong. The men took him to the police station and threatened to lock him up in a cell and charge him with possession of fraudulent documents or he should pay three thousand naira (N3,000) that's about eleven pounds seventy seven pence (£11.77p). Because he needed to get out of police trouble and apply for his visa he took them to the cash point and withdrew the money and gave it to them and they allowed him to leave. That's the case in Nigeria, bribery and corruption is found within the police. Sometimes some innocent people have been put in prison for crime they know nothing about just because they could offer no bribe.

Simon applied for the first time for a UK visa in 2007. He was stopped again by two men the second time and the same thing happened again and they collected money from him before they would let him go. He just had to go that's why he paid them that money to let him go if not he wondered what would have happened to him at the police station. In May 2007, he received a phone call from the British Embassy that he should attend an interview a week after and he should come with some documents.

Simon told his friend whom he was living with because he was supposed to live with his married aunty who lived in London when he arrived in the UK. In May 2007, he went to the British High Commission at Walter Carrington Crescent, Victoria Island, Lagos and he was interviewed. At the end of the day he was granted a Student visa that ran for 16 months. He was very happy when he left the embassy. He called Mr Dimka and told him and went to his house to show him the visa. He was dumbfounded and said how can he get a visa on a virgin passport? But at the end of the day he congratulated him. When he got home he showed it to his friend he lived with and he was very happy and informed his aunty about it.

That night he received several calls about twenty five times from his younger siblings saying their mother is dying and there was nothing anybody can do and that he should come quickly. He didn't sleep throughout that night because of the calls. He left where he was living with his friend at 5am at Lawanson, Surulere to go to Badagry on getting where his mother was, he met her dead and he was told that she died within minutes before he arrived. He met his two siblings, aunty and others crying. His aunty asked him why he wasted time before he came that maybe if he were around she would have lived and his siblings were telling him that she was asking to see him before she died. His siblings told him also that she was struggling for breath and wanted to say something before she died but it seemed that she was choking.

Simon's mother died a day after he got his visa to come to the UK. She never knew or lived to see his visa before she died. She was taken to Badagry mortuary on the day she died by himself, his younger brother Jason and their elder sister's husband Mr Olusegun Obafemi. His mother was buried a week after her death in June 2007 in a cemetery at Mowo along Badagry expressway. Mr Dimka helped to contribute money towards the casket and money for the mortuary expenses. The loss of Simon's mother dealt a very big blow to him and his younger siblings. At that time they lost their only hope of survival because she has been there for them all the time.

The day Simon's mother was buried, His mother's family called for a meeting to reunite all the children. His elder sister Ruth and his elder brother Henry always cooperate between each other they never liked their mother at a point until her death and they have been speaking evil about Simon especially and his younger siblings. Simon's elder brother Henry was reported many times to be a cult member, even his elder sister Ruth confirmed it from sources. The meeting that day did not resolve anything as expected because there were so many denials and pretence as if things were alright. His mother before she died has always called for peace and reconciliation between all her children and said they should forgive one another and also forgive her if she has hurt any one of them.

Because of his elder brother's evil intentions towards Simon, his uncle Franklin, his mother's younger brother told him to leave where he was living with his friend at Lawanson and move to live in his apartment with his kids because Henry can't be trusted since he was a member of a secret cult society and he has never liked Simon developing hatred for him and speaking evil about him and always looking for every opportunity to harm him. He left his friend's apartment and went to live with his uncle and his kids. His uncle lived alone in Port Harcourt in the Southern part of Nigeria but his kids lived at Orile Iganmu in Lagos. He comes once in a while to visit them. During this period Simon often felt the presence of his mother as if she was watching him. Sometimes he dreamt about her and not just her but his elder brother Charlie who died years back. At this time he was not normal mentally but no one noticed it not even himself. He still did everyday tasks and related and talked to people normally but deep within him he hallucinated on most occasions and heard voices which are persecutory and frightening. At this time he would always feel he had special powers and thought someone was reading his thoughts or taking his thoughts away. At this time he started believing there were some evil forces against him which may be from his family members who doesn't want his progress and he should always pray and go to Church to protect myself. He always felt his elder brother and sister were plotting for his downfall.

Simon was still visiting Mr Dimka from time to time helping by running errands for his office but he never knew exactly what his company was all about because he never revealed or let him know or get involve in his business or close to knowing what his business entails or does. He was only told to always maybe post a letter in a while or just sit in the office watching TV or checking his email and chatting with his friends online. Mr Dimka helped him a lot and when it was getting close to time when he was to travel he gave Simon one hundred thousand naira (N100,000) that's about four hundred pounds (£400) for his flight to London.

There was a girl Simon like at that time they both served together during his NYSC programme. He had already told my Dimka about her earlier. He called Simon on the phone one day and asked for the girl's number because he wanted to employ her because his secretary was not serious and he couldn't depend on her because she had told him that she is not happy doing the job. So Simon gave him the girl's number and he later called her to tell her that Mr Dimka will call her and he wants to offer her a job. She was very happy and told her mother about it. But later Simon started feeling uneasy, so he called Mr Dimka's secretary to enquiry why she wants to leave the job, but she told him that she and Mr Dimka have not discussed anything to that extent and their relationship as an employee and employer was intact and everything was alright. The way she sounded on the phone Simon could sense she was not happy. She then told him that she will ask Mr Dimka what the problem was and find out why he wants to sack her and bring in another person.
At this time Simon then realised that Mr Dimka was up to something. He started to ponder over this things and he got so paranoid that he called Mr Dimka's secretary on the phone to meet up somewhere. When they met he told her that he was going to kill Mr Dimka. Meanwhile Mr Dimka's driver has blamed Simon for giving that girl's number to Mr Dimka and he has warned Simon earlier that whatever he tells the secretary or that girl that they will go to tell Mr Dimka because he is a rich man and told Simon that Nigerian ladies can do anything for money.
The secretary went to tell Mr Dimka that Simon called her on phone and told him everything he had said about him. At this time Simon lost respect for Mr Dimka. That girl eventually went to see Mr Dimka and when she came back, he asked her what they discussed

concerning the job he wants to offer her but she said nothing really that she doesn't even know what he does and he was just talking about his wife and kids and the places he has travelled, that they didn't talk about anything like employment and she told Simon that Mr Dimka was asking her what type of person he was and if they were dating. Simon advised her not to go to Mr Dimka again and he doesn't trust him and he really doesn't know the type of business he is running because he hides everything he does. She agreed and said she will never pick his call next time he calls.

Simon stopped calling Mr Dimka after that time. The day he was meant to travel his younger brother Jason and Sister Hannah were with him. They had come a week earlier to live with him at their uncle's apartment. His cousins told him that the landlady of the house has told them that there are too many people living in the house, so therefore they will have to move out of the apartment or his younger siblings should move out. When he heard this he was in distress so was his younger siblings. There was no where they could move to, so he decided to speak to the landlady's son to help talk to his mother to allow his younger siblings stay with their cousins because they have nowhere to go and their mother just died. When the landlady's son heard this he was very upset and he told him that they should go together to talk to his mother. When they got to his mother, he asked his mother why she said such a thing. She replied that she has never uttered such a statement and she asked someone to call his cousins to her presence and there she asked both of them when she ever said such thing. They replied that, that's what their father ordered them to say, that he said he only allowed Simon to come and stay for a short time and not his other siblings. At this time they were so angry and disappointed. Simon then begged his cousins to allow his siblings to stay with them for a short time and when he get to London and started working he will send money for them to get their own apartment.

Simon left Nigeria in September, 2007 at around 10pm on a flight that had stopped over at Schiphol airport in Amsterdam and had a connected flight from there to London. Meanwhile his younger brother Jason, his friend whom he stayed with for a short time after his NYSC service Emeka and that girl followed him to Murtala International airport in Lagos, Nigeria. Since he left Nigeria till this day he have never stepped his foot there. Simon arrived the UK in September, 2007, at Heathrow airport in London after stopping over at Schiphol Airport in Amsterdam because he took flight from Murtala International Airport in Lagos. His friend's aunt's husband came to pick him up. Meanwhile his travelling to the UK was kept secret from other members of his family even from his father. His friend's in-law was a very nice man, his name was Mr Mogaji. He is a Nigerian from the Yoruba ethnic group.

Simon has had so many people who have helped him one way or the other. When he was about to travel to the UK, his childhood friend Mr Omobola Tyson gave him a travelling bag to put his belongings in and he gave him twenty thousand naira (N20,000) that's about seventy eight pounds and forty three pence (£78.43p). Even one of his other friends Mr Osareme Eguabor gave him five thousand naira (N5,000) that's about nineteen pounds and sixty one pence (£19.61p). One of his father's aunt's Mrs Henrieta Oboro gave him fifteen thousand naira (N15,000) that's about fifty eight pounds and eighty two pence (£58.82p) and his uncle Mr Franklin Akpan had given him ten thousand naira earlier (N10,000) that's about thirty nine pounds and twenty two pence (£39.22p). Simon came to the UK with only £50 because he gave the rest of the money to his siblings.

Simon and Mr Mogaji stayed at the airport for a few minutes and he bought him snacks and coffee on that morning, that was when he felt the cold of Europe. He bought him a train travel card for that day and they went home. When they got home he introduced him to his kids and he met his wife, his friend's aunt. The family he lived with this time were Joseph the eldest who was 16 at the time, Charmaine who was 14 and the youngest Amy who was 10.

CHAPTER FOUR
MY FIRST PSYCHIATRY EPISODE

When Simon got to London he called his friend to tell him he arrived safely and he also called his younger siblings but they had bad news that day, they told him that their cousins have driven them out of the house and they were in the street. His younger sister was with her 9 months old baby at that time. Simon was under pressure to get a job at that time so he could help his siblings. He told them to go to their aunt's house to stay there for a while until he started a job and would be able to send them money. Meanwhile he only had a student visa at that time and he was only permitted to work only 20 hours a week as a student under law. Many people from less developed countries often come to developed countries for a better life and to help themselves and their family. He was unable to go to school because he had no sponsor, so he was left with the option of looking for a job to care for himself and go to school later and be able to qualify to work full time, live in the UK and then help his siblings. He was under serious pressure because he got calls every day about the situation of his younger siblings.

The first month of his arrival he saw peace like he have never experienced before. Things were blooming but the situation about his siblings kept worrying him. In October 2007, he met a former classmate called James Ariwolo in Woolwich. He was very surprised to see him; he was born in the UK but grew up in Nigeria. Simon told him that he was looking for a job and he told him that he can help him get a job. He told him to expect a call from his younger brother the next day and they would take him to a place where he can work "underground" in a sandwich factory in Bromley-by bow in East London.

Meanwhile James was a full time student at that time; he was studying chemical engineering at London South Bank University. He told Simon that he will be working with someone else's documents bearing the name Ademosu Ariwolo but that was his documents, he was not been smart enough at that time to realise that he will be working with his own friend's document and not someone else's. Because he was so desperate for a job at that time and would do anything to earn a living, he saw the desperation in him and he told him that he will be paying 30% of his earnings every week after tax to the owner of the document because he had spoken to the person and the person agreed. Though he said initially the person said he will be paying 40% after tax every week but he spoke with the owner of the document and that he was his classmate in secondary school so he should reduce the percentage. Simon was meant to be working from 6am to 3pm daily Monday through Friday with an hour break.

When Simon got home he told his friend's aunty husband Mr Mogaji, he was not very happy about it. He told him that it was cheating. But he said there was nothing he could do about it but the choice was his, so he had to decide but he wouldn't advise him to take up that offer he said. The next day he received a phone call from James' younger brother and he told him to meet him at Woolwich in Southeast London. Simon met him where he asked him to and he took him to the factory and told him that he should get prepared the next morning and be at the factory at 6am. He told Simon how he should sign the timesheet in and out before and after work hours and told him to stay away from people from work, that he should never relate with anyone especially Nigerians and should not tell anyone anything concerning his immigration status. Though that time he was not living in the UK as an illegal immigrant because he still had a valid visa but he was not allowed to work more than 20 hours a week since he had a student visa. Simon woke up at 3am the next day got prepared and left for work in the cold. He got to the work and worked for 6 days but the supervisor dropped some workers after six days because the department where he worked got shut down for a few days. he was supposed to get his pay for 6 days but James paid him only for 3 days, telling him that he didn't submit the timesheet and the Agency whom he was working with said they only saw attendance for only 3 days and that was the amount they paid and he had already deducted the 30% they agreed on before he took up the job. This brought a quarrel between Simon and him and they had fallout, till this day he has not seen him and he had lost contact with him. Simon used the money he got from the job to buy himself some food and other essential items like toiletries and some clothes. At this time his mental state had started deteriorating and getting worse than when he was in Nigeria. Most times he use to perceive people around him whom others can't see and he get personal messages from reading the newspaper or listening to the TV.

One day he was walking in the street and someone gave him a leaflet inviting him to attend a Pentecostal Church in Woolwich. He attended one Thursday because they do hold several mid-week services in different locations in member's homes. The people were very friendly and one of them was a solicitor and he helped him got a job through an Agency working with the Royal Mail in Sydenham in Southeast London. He had the job just for 3 days he couldn't cope because of his mental state and the demands of the job. At this time he started having trouble with the family he lives with, he couldn't understand what was happening to him at the time. He started hallucinating and suspecting the family he was living with, if they have had contacts with Mr Dimka and if they are trying to manipulate his brain. He got so paranoid that he wrote an email to Mr Dimka accusing him of killing his mother and taking the girl that he loved. Mr Dimka replied him with aggression asking if he is hallucinating and what must have brought about the email he sent him. He replied to him again telling him not to deny it that he must have killed his mother. At this time he couldn't control it because he heard voices commanding him and sometimes it was persecutory and he tried to talk back within himself to challenge this voice sometimes.

Then Mr Dimka's daughter Edith replied to him through an email insulting him and bringing the instances where his elder brother Henry have been a fraudulent person when he was living with them some time ago and saying, why should Simon accuse someone who has helped him get to the UK and that why is he repaying good with evil. But Simon replied to her saying that her father is evil and he killed his mother and she should go find out properly what her father does in secret. At this time neither Mr Dimka nor his daughter replied to Simon again.
Simon's mental state deteriorated to the extent that he couldn't take care of his personal hygiene. There was a day Mr Mogaji told him that his 10-year-old daughter reported that he was singing love songs to her and he warned him that if she ever goes to the police to report him, he would be in trouble. Simon got angry because nothing like that has ever happened. He sings songs in the house which were Nigerian songs and which the kids don't understand at that time, so it might be that she was around when he was singing so she thought those songs was intended for her since those songs was not in English. At this time, his friend's aunt started telling him to look for somewhere else to stay. Every day that passes by Mr Mogaji tells him that he is worried about his mental state and he would have to leave their home. At that time Simon had no friends, relatives or did not

know anyone he could live with. He started withdrawing from everyone in the house, He would stay alone in the room given to him and not come out until everyone had gone out. He started receiving phone calls from his friend Emeka and his mother from Nigeria telling him that they have been having complaints about him. They said they had known him to be a very quiet and shy person when he was in Nigeria, that they know him fully well that he can't just change suddenly. They were so concerned and asked Simon what problems he was having but he couldn't point out what his problem was to them, all he said was that he is innocent and they just want him out of their house.

Not long after Simon was told to leave the house by his friend's aunt and he ended up in the streets of London with all his belongings. That night he roamed the streets of London looking for a place to sleep. As he was walking the streets he kept pondering in his mind what was really going on with him. He started to imagine his life of being a graduate from Nigeria and being in the UK with no home. Simon started thinking what kind of life he was going to live from that moment. As he was walking in the street a girl was sharing a Christian leaflet and he collected a leaflet from her, and when he looked at the address it was a Redeem Christian Church of
GOD. So he went to the Church. Luckily for him there were just finishing the service. So he waited for a few minutes and thinking what to do. At first he was thinking of going to talk to the head of the Church. But he summoned courage because he was too timid to talk to anyone he saw, so he approached a man and he told him briefly his story and asked if he could assist him with a temporal accommodation. He asked him where Simon was from and he asked him if he was living in the UK illegally, Simon told him where he was from and told him he just came into the UK a few months ago and had a visa that is valid for another year and he showed him the

documentary proof. He told him that he could only assist him with an accommodation for two weeks only because where he was living belongs to his elder brother and his elder brother comes once in a while to the house because he works outside London. He was very relieved when he told him he could help him for a short time. He took him into his house and introduced him to his wife and other brothers. He had his shower and he was provided with food to eat. This Christian man really helped him, he assisted him in getting his first provisional driver's licence and he helped him secure a temporary job working in a sandwich company in Orpington in Kent. At this time his mental state has deteriorated further. He started sensing people where watching him and knew his every moves. He thought people could read his thoughts. When he read newspapers he got personal messages and would think the news was referring to him. He started showing complete symptoms of Paranoid Schizophrenia.

This was a very dreadful experience for him. At this time he didn't know what was wrong with him. When it was two weeks he couldn't get an alternative place to move to so the man gave him one more week to enable him to get a place. But meanwhile he started sending text messages to his boss about what was going on in his head. Whenever he started having the symptoms he would send it straight to his boss, for example when he hear "you are going to die" he will send it to her phone and when he replied in his head to the voice that he is not going to die he would send it as well to her. She became scared of him and called him to her office and asking what was the meaning of all the messages he have been sending her. He told her that those are the messages he just wanted to tell her that he hears voices telling him everything he have sent to her so far and told her to be afraid of some of her employers. After that day she stopped him from coming to work that was how he lost his job.

At the end of the extra one week given to Simon to look for a place, He still didn't get enough money to rent a place of his own and he had lost his job. So he was told to leave because his symptoms affected him to the extent that he started picking up quarrels with every member of the house where he lived. Before he left he stopped talking to anyone. That night he went to Queen Mary Hospital in Sidcup, Kent, and looked for a safe place where he left his belongings and he went to sleep under the cold with no cover close to one of the wards. He could not sleep for a long time because of the cold. He woke up in the middle of the night and roamed about the Hospital until it was around 3am. He left the Hospital and walked a distance of about 10 miles and came across a cab office, he went in there to stay for a while just to get warmth. When it was dawn, he went to where he left his belongings but couldn't find them. This was around 9am. He had left his belongings close to an entrance where there was a door. So he knocked at the door and a man opened and asked him what he wanted. Meanwhile there were about eight to nine people in the room when the man opened the door. He told him that he left his bag at the entrance to the door but couldn't find it and asked if he saw it. He told him to come in and he was greeted by other people in the room. They asked him questions about how he came to leave his bag, what was inside the bag and his name. He told them everything. They all felt very sorry for him and the bag was handed to him. They have seen the bag and kept it and wondering who must have left a bag with important documents in it. The bag contains his Passport with a valid visa, Birth Certificate, Family photos and his baby photos, His University Certificate, NYSC Certificate, Secondary School Certificates and examination results.

He was very happy when he was given the bag and he thanked them and bid them goodbye.

So he left the Hospital that day and he could remember it was Sunday 23rd December 2007. He left and was roaming the streets of London again in the cold. The cold was very severe that he was moving from one store to another staying for some minutes in one store before he moved again as he walked just to get warm. So he came across a Methodist Church at Plumstead Common in Southeast London and waited at the door because the door was shut. The service starts at 11am and he got there around 10am. So he waited in the cold for one hour before the door was opened. He went to the Church because he had thought in his heart that he could get help in terms of accommodation. He attended the service and met friendly people and he received a warm welcome at the end of the service and had coffee and biscuits for breakfast.

At the end of the service he approached a Christian brother and told him that he was homeless and needed a place to stay. He told him that there is a homeless winter shelter for the homeless in Islington North London and he volunteered to take him there in his car. He drove him after the service, as he drove he fell asleep in the car because it was so comfortable and warm but when he woke up they were at City Road in Islington the venue of the homeless shelter. The Christian Brother shook his hand and said hope he enjoy his stay at the homeless centre and he bid him goodbye.

Simon joined the queue and waited for some hours before he got entrance into the building. They were searched and their belongings were kept in a safe place and they were given a tag to wear on their wrist. The tag was meant for identification in case they go outside the building and when returning they will have to show it as proof that they have been in the building before. During this time in the homeless shelter his mental health have fallen so bad, the symptoms becomes increasing every day. Simon could remember on Tuesday 25th December Christmas day when Her Majesty Queen Elizabeth II was addressing the UK and the commonwealth countries he heard a voice telling him that he came from the Royal family in England and he want to return to the Palace. Simon perceived at that time that only the Queen can save him from all the troubles he was facing at that time.

Meanwhile the homeless shelter was supposed to be open from Sunday 23rd December till Sunday 30th December 2007. At that time Simon was just wondering where else he would go to after the shelter closes. As he was pondering, he saw a beautiful blonde haired lady who was a member of staff for the homeless shelter and he asked to speak with her. They were just chatting and she gave him her email ID if he wants to contact her. The next day he saw her he told her that she should marry him because he fears going back to Nigeria and that he hears voices wanting to kill him. He told her about Mr Dimka but she told him that she can't marry him and she introduced him to her father and mother because they were all volunteering in the homeless shelter. Her name was Leona Andrews. She told her father all what he had told her and her father sat him down and advised him and told him that marriage is not the way out of his problem that the best way to solve his problem is to solve any problem he have with Mr Dimka and then claim Asylum if he has a profound fear of returning to Nigeria. At this time Simon was disappointed and he didn't see her again till this day. When it was getting to the end of his stay at the homeless shelters, some rough sleepers were applying for an accommodation through the local council but because he was not entitled to it at that time he couldn't apply. There was a man he met at the shelter; his name was Stephen he works with the social services. His father was a Nigerian and his mother from Guyana. He spoke with him about his situation he advised him to throw away all his belongings including his passport and all other documents he has. Because he was paranoid he obeyed him. That was how he lost his family photos, baby photos, his university certificate, passport and all other documents. He told Simon that he was going to help him get his legal right in the UK but he would have to be patient because it will take a bit time. He advised him to live ''underground'' and keep a low profile. He gave Simon his business address and said he can come in anytime for a course because the social services run courses for the homeless and those on benefit.

Simon left the shelter in the morning of Wednesday 31st December 2007 because the place was shut. He roamed the streets of London once again in the very cold winter. He received a leaflet where he can find Islington Cold Weather Shelter from the homeless centre he left. The Islington Cold Weather Shelter runs from 1st January till 31st March every year at that time. So he spent the night in the streets roaming about and taking Bus from one end where it leaves to the last stop where it terminates and he would repeat it again to the other end just to get warm. At many occasions he fell asleep and the driver had to wake him up to tell me that the Bus is at the last stop.

The Islington Cold Weather Shelter is a shelter for the homeless during the winter period for homeless people around Islington in North London. It is organised by the Church of England in different places around the borough of Islington. Each borough in London has a winter shelter for the homeless in London. On the 1st January 2008, Simon was queuing up in a very long queue waiting for the doors to open in one of the designated Churches. The door was finally opened around 8pm and they all went in. He was lucky to get a bed space that night because they were too many and the spaces were quickly filled up. Others who couldn't get a bed space were given food and drink and referred to other centres for the night shelter.

Each day of the week he slept in different cold weather shelters and he got food and drink and provided with a bed space only during the night. During the day he roamed about the streets of London. Sometimes he did go to restaurants and he would eat from the remnants or leftovers from other people. He became so unwell and lost so much weight. At this time he heard voices telling him he will die and also heard voices commanding him to get prepared because he will get attacked. Simon's mental state deteriorated to the point the keeper of the homeless shelter started observing him and at that time he was a concern. He called him one day and was questioning him. He asked him where he was from and how he got into the UK. Simon told him everything about his life and he told him that he is going to refer him to a Psychiatrist and a social worker but he told him that there was nothing wrong with him that he was fine. He told him he need to see a Psychiatrist and he must meet with one, so he gave him an address and phone number to contact for the next day when he leaves the shelter.
The next day Simon left the shelter and he heard the voice again which he used to hear telling him to go to the library to attack anyone he sees. He heeded to the voice and he walked to a library about 2 miles away. He went up to the First floor where there were many people reading and he attacked a young lady who was with a laptop. He threw her laptop to the floor and he pushed her and she staggered backwards and screamed shouting "get off me". He held her and squeezed her tight, she screamed for help while the other people in the library ran away.

The security came and separated him from the lady, they brought him to the ground and held him to the ground and called the police and the ambulance. When the paramedics came they took his blood sample and took him into the ambulance and decided to take him to the Hospital. On his way to the Hospital they were asking if he was married he said yes and his wife was Leona Andrews the girl he met at the homeless shelter centre. They asked him where he lives he told them in the streets. They asked him if he was from Ghana he said yes then they asked him what his name was he said Amoah. So they got to Whittington Hospital in Archway in North London in the borough of Islington. He was asked what his name was by the staff in the Hospital so they could locate his file but he told them Amoah and they asked for his surname he told them he had no surname. So he was taken to a room and he waited there for some minutes and he was given food to eat and later a Doctor came to attend to him. The Doctor was asking him his name he told him Amoah but no surname. Then he asked him what brought him to the Hospital he explained to him he heard a voice telling him to go to the library to attack someone so he obeyed. He asked him, how he attacked her. He told him he threw her laptop to the floor and grabbed her, pulled her hair and squeezed her tight. Then he told him to go and wished him luck. At that time he heard the voice again telling him that the Doctor approved what he have done to the innocent young girl and he was safe. But he kept imagining what was wrong with him and why he attacked the young lady, he kept wondering if he was sane and he kept telling himself that his name is Amoah and he was from Ghana not Nigeria.

That night Simon went to the cold weather shelter and the keeper of the shelter asked him how was his appointment with the social service workers he told him he didn't go for any appointment and told him what had happened that day. He felt so sorry for him and he told him he must go the next day. The next day he booked the appointment on his behalf and he went to see the social service workers. When he got there, he was given a seat to sit and a Psychiatrist and other social service workers were asking him questions. He told them he used to hear voices commanding him to do things and he never obeyed only the day before when he actually went into the library to attack a young lady. They told Simon that he had to go with them to Hospital so they can arrange an admission for him. They asked him what he thought. But because he wanted to get off the streets he agreed to be taken into Hospital. He never knew he had mental illness at that time. He was just thinking of the comfort of a new home. He told them that he was not going to stay in the Hospital for long and they agreed with him.

So Simon's first admission in Hospital was at St Pancras Hospital, in King's Cross, in North London in the borough of Camden this was in January 2008. There he was diagnosed by Dr Jude Moss from the University College London and his illness was Paranoid Schizophrenia. That was how he came to know that his condition was a mental illness at that time. So he was detained in hospital under the mental health act.

CHAPTER FIVE
MY DISCHARGE AND SECOND PSYCHIATRY EPISODE

Simon remained in the Psychiatry Hospital receiving treatment. There was a ward round every Monday and Friday whereby the doctors always saw patients to monitor their progress. Simon could remember his first ward round he was telling Dr Moss that Nigerians wants to kill him and he was born in Sri Lanka. He also gave him a piece of paper where he wrote messages about Mr Dimka and Nigeria. He wrote in the piece of paper that Mr Dimka wants to kill him and there are so many Nigerians who will kill him if he goes back to the country. He could not remember anything more he had said at that time. When he was in hospital, Ben Collins was the primary nurse allocated to him, he was from Cameroon and he was a very good psychiatric nurse. During Simon's time in hospital Dr Moss booked an appointment for him, so a Forensic Psychiatric Doctor came into the ward to interview him because of the incident that occurred in the library. The police had wanted to come and interview Simon but because he was not mentally fit for an interview Dr Moss kept them at bay until he was fit enough.

In April 2008, the police came to arrest Simon on in the ward in connection with the incident that happened at the library. The hospital got him a solicitor and Ben Collins followed him to the police station. At the police station his finger print were taken and a swab was taken from his mouth and a photo was taken of his face. Then he was put in the cell for some hours. He was later brought out and taken to see his solicitor and his psychiatric nurse. Simon's solicitor interviewed him and told him questions he will be asked by the police and how to answer them. Then they were called into the interview room by two police officers and he was interviewed in the presence of his solicitor and his psychiatric nurse. At the interview they asked him to describe what happened that day. Simon was able to explain to them all that happened that day. They asked Simon how he felt that moment during the interview, and he told them that he was really sorry for what had happened and said it was due to his illness and that he never had the intention of assaulting anyone but that was his first episode he had of his illness. At the end of the interview he was taken back to the cell to wait for their decision.

After some hours they brought Simon out and gave him a caution and gave him a copy and he was released. Simon's solicitor told him that it will remain in the record for five years until then it will be taken off. So he went back to the hospital with his nurse. Meanwhile he was well enough to be discharged from hospital a few weeks after the police came to arrest him, but because he have nowhere to go he was kept in the hospital.

Christine Baker from the Early Intervention Service, which is a specialist mental health team in Camden and Islington borough of London, had come to see him earlier in the ward to discuss how they can be of support in terms of getting him accommodation. In June 2008, the Islington no recourse to public funds panel team agreed to support Simon with accommodation. They got him a studio flat in the borough of Islington. Simon was discharged from hospital in June 2008, after staying in hospital for almost six months. His rent was being paid for by the Islington council and they supported him with subsistence every week towards feeding since he wasn't entitled to receive benefit at that time.

Simon stayed at that address and he continued to see his care coordinator every week who was Christine Baker at that time to monitor his mental state. Simon made two friends while he was in the hospital, Friday Timilehin who was a Nigerian born British citizen and also Grace Anifowoshe who was a British citizen. They were patients in the hospital at that time with him. Simon had now lost contact with them. Simon continued taking his medication at that time until after sometime. He felt very well and strong so he decided to stop taking his medication around September 2008.

In September 2008 Simon was employed by A.E.A/S.O.S Ltd which was a cleaning company. He was posted to work at a Primary School in Archway just 15mins walk from where he lived at that time in North London. At this time he was living well and happy but he didn't tell his care coordinator that he had stopped taking his medication. Simon spent the Christmas and New Year alone in his flat that year. He did wake up at 4:30am to go to work because he resumes at 5am and finish at 8am. He made friends with his neighbours Tim Gary whose father was a Jamaican and his mother was a Ghanaian though he was born in the UK. He also made friends with Kelly Philips. Tim was a schizophrenic patient so was Kelly. They had both just come out of prison at the time and were given temporary accommodation by the Islington council.

When Simon's visa was running out towards the end of 2008, he applied through the Early Intervention Service to the Home Office to extend his visa and his care coordinator gave him a letter to support his application. He applied on health and compassionate grounds so that his visa could be extended but the mistake he made in the application was applying for an indefinite leave to remain in the UK. In February 2009, the Home Office replied to Simon's application rejecting it giving reasons that he had applied outside the UK immigration rules and the secretary of state is not willing to exercise her discretion to extending his leave to remain in the UK, so therefore he had 28 days to leave the UK or face deportation to Nigeria by the Home Office or if he have any reason for him to be permitted by the immigration authority which he had not stated before then he should do so within 28 days of receiving the letter. At that time his legal right in the UK had expired two months earlier. That was how he faced another battle. Simon called a Christian brother, Thomas Matthew an immigration solicitor whom he had known when he just moved into the UK and he booked an appointment for him to see him that same day. Fortunately for Simon it was a Thursday when they hold Christian fellowship service in his house. So he went to meet him that day he prayed with him and he told him to go see a solicitor in his borough who deals with legal aid clients. He said he works for a firm of solicitors and he would not be able to take up his case because his firm doesn't deal with legal aid so a legal aid solicitor would be the best option for him. So Simon went to search for a legal aid solicitor through the citizen advice bureau and he saw a solicitor in Islington borough. He made appointment to see one solicitor from the Islington Law Centre, her name was Sheena Jacob.

Simon was able to see her a few days after and when he saw her, she interviewed him and asked him questions about how he got to the UK, his family history, where he has been living. She also asked him why he feared returning to Nigeria. She then ran assessment to see if he qualified for a legal aid service. At the end of the assessment she told him that she is willing to take up his case but he had a very slim chance of winning the case because she told him that he should have sought legal advice or applied through a solicitor when he made his first application. She also told him that the only way he could get his legal status in the UK was to apply for discretionary leave to remain or exceptional leave to remain. She also told him that she would need a Psychiatry report from his Psychiatric Doctor.

Meanwhile Simon had already told her that his family in Nigeria have disowned him because he had a mental illness. This was what his friends Grace and Friday advised him to say to the solicitor if not she would not be able to help him. Sheena Jacob took up Simon's case and she filed an appeal to the Immigration Tribunal. Simon was sent a letter to come for his hearing in April 2009.

Simon's solicitor Sheena Jacob was at the immigration tribunal before him on that day and before the hearing started she explained to him the process and advised him not to say anything unless he was been asked a question by the judge. Within minutes the appeal started and the judge was asking Simon's solicitor some questions about his application. The solicitor from the Home Office told the judge that since he have overstayed his visa he have no right to remain in the UK and he said what's the proof that his family have disowned him and he also said he have families in Nigeria and not in the UK so therefore he should return there where he will get treatment he also said that from findings which he had done and research there is adequate treatment for Psychiatric disorders in Nigeria he also stressed that Simon have no strong ties in the UK and stressed that the UK government will not be willing to allow him to live on state hand-outs even supposing if they decided to grant him a leave to remain. He then turned to Simon and asked him what will he do if he was granted a visa to remain in the UK? Simon told him that he will find part-time work to do in his field of study while he fully recovered from his illness then he will go to study for his Masters to make contribution to the UK.

Then Simon's solicitor was allowed to speak. She told the judge that the Home Office solicitor said Simon have overstayed his visa so therefore should be deported.
She said in response to that, Simon applied to extend his visa not after his visa was expired but before it expired so it is of no basis by him to mention that. His solicitor produced a copy of Simon's friend (Grace) data page of her passport and a copy of evidence of her travel to Nigeria few weeks before that time, to the judge at that moment saying she actually went to Nigeria for a visit and was at Simon's family's house and told them everything that had happened to him in the UK. Grace actually travelled to Nigeria to visit her own family on holiday so Simon was very lucky at that time that she went to Nigeria and the evidence was presented to the judge by his solicitor. On the issue of state hand-outs Simon's solicitor stressed that from his Psychiatry report, Simon's Psychiatry doctor have stressed that he should remain on his medication for a long period of time while regular meeting with his care coordinator is closely monitored and also get him involved on social activities through the occupational therapist. She then asked why the authorities would then allow him to go back to Nigeria when all these services are lacking and she provided evidences about mental health services to the judge. She also said that though he had no family of his own in the UK but he has made some reasonable and quite close friends while in the UK which in the future can be his family and also why can't he be given the opportunity to live like every other human and would one day have a family of his own.

The solicitor was again given the opportunity to speak again and he said, from the doctor's report she never mentioned anything about any suicidal attempt by Simon then why mentioning it in Simon's solicitor's report? Simon's solicitor responded that he had decided to make it a secret but only confided in her to tell her about it. The judge responded that why should Simon have confided in her since he have only known her for a brief period of time compared to his Psychiatry doctor or his care coordinator whom he had known longer and had contact with almost every week. The judge then said, Simon has only been in the UK for not up to two years at that time and he have not really had a family life in the UK, so those are what will be considered plus other factors when making a judgement like for example she said Simon's mental illness started while in Nigeria not in the UK and things must have changed in Nigeria at the present compared to when his elder brother died in 2003. Then she asked if there are any more things to say by either parties or any evidences to submit.

Simon's solicitor asked for the judge to give her more time to get an additional report from his Psychiatry Doctor, Dr Candy Woods to clarify the issue of the case of a suicidal attempt if he will be sent back to Nigeria but the judge refused, saying an additional time cannot be granted. So she closed the hearing. The hearing took almost two hours on that day.

After the hearing Simon's immigration solicitor told him that the case is now in the hands of the judge and the court will make a decision normally within two weeks. Simon and his solicitor left the court that day and went to catch a train that took them from the outskirts of London close to Heathrow airport to north London. When they got to the Borough of Islington he bided Simon goodbye and he went home.

At this time Simon's mental state has started deteriorating again. Anytime he feels like he is having the symptoms he would quickly take the antipsychotics and when he starts to feel better he would stop taking it again. That was how he lived at that time. He didn't go out at all; he remained indoors all the time thinking about his life. Sometimes he did go to visit his friends Grace or Friday whom he met in the hospital. They always encouraged him and they took him like a brother. Simon is a very quiet person, he doesn't talk much but he is a very good listener. He doesn't socialise much because he gets depressed and experiences social withdrawal symptoms. That is why the early intervention service organised a film group once in a month and badminton group every Monday to meet up with people and exercise to cope with the side effects of his medication.

Some of the major side effects he had when taking Risperidone was muscle stiffness, frequency in urinating, blurred vision, weight gain, swollen eyes and lips and constipation. Most times in the morning he finds it very hard to get out of bed, he couldn't just do some normal work like bending down, touching his feet with his fingers. It was very serious so he had to complain to his Care Coordinator who always booked him an appointment to see his Psychiatrist. Simon's Psychiatrist reduced the dose of his medication at that time from 4mg to 3mg to monitor the side effects. He felt better at that time. But still he wasn't taking the medication frequently.
After two weeks the immigration tribunal upheld the decision to grant Simon leave to remain in the UK. Simon's immigration solicitor called him on the phone to tell him the news. This affected him psychologically. He stopped eating because he lost appetite and lost weight. His mental state became more unstable at that time. All he did that time was to inform his care coordinator how he felt. She would encourage him and book him in frequently to more groups just to take his mind off the current situation but it didn't really work well with him because he wasn't taking his medication as he should but he never told her. Simon's immigration status that time was the key to his mental state because he couldn't go to school, work legally and live in the UK at that time. Simon's immigration solicitor then told him that she is

going to appeal on his behalf, so he doesn't need to do anything. She had already told him that he have a very slim chance of succeeding in his application but she said all fingers crossed she will try her best to make sure she put in for a good appeal. Simon's immigration solicitor put in for the appeal on his behalf and he waited for some time around a month before he received another decision this time the court upheld the decision again asking him to return to Nigeria to get treatment and also said his Psychiatrist didn't mention in her report any case of suicidal attempt so therefore they can't consider his appeal based on that.

Simon's immigration solicitor then told him that he had exhausted every right of his appeal except just one last chance which is to apply to the European Higher Court of Law. And she told him that will take up to four to six months before a final decision will be made. So she told him to relax and have his fingers crossed and she will help him make the appeal and then they will wait to see what the final decision would be. At this time it was around June 2009. So Simon's immigration solicitor made the final appeal to the European Higher Court of Law while he waited for the final decision.

Meanwhile he was so scared that the final appeal will not go through, he started looking for other alternatives like maybe get a partner or get someone to marry because the judge had said he had no family life in the UK. Also his friends have been telling him that he need to search for a woman to start a relationship with and probably have a child. Simon was really under pressure at that time. One day he went to visit his friend Friday who lives at King's Cross St Pancras in central London, on getting there, he saw him throwing away his friend Badejo's belongings out of his apartment because Badejo was living with him at that time. He asked what had happened. He told Simon that Badejo was spying on him and reading his personal letters, going through his bank letters and copying contacts from his phone and he said Badejo refused to pay or contribute towards the bills in the house. So because of that he is sending him out to go live elsewhere. Badejo denied all the accusations. But because Simon felt pity for Badejo and he said he hasn't got anywhere to put his belongings and to sleep for the night, Simon secretly called him aside to tell him to move to live with him. He didn't want Friday to know because that might not be good for their relationship or he might tell him not to help him. Simon knows Friday very well and he is a very good friend and Badejo is someone he know through Friday and he told him he graduated from the University Simon went to in Nigeria.

Simon helped Badejo move his bags and other properties into his studio flat. Badejo started living with Simon from then. Then Simon told him about his situation about how he came to the UK, all what he had been through and the situation about his immigration. Badejo told Simon that he can help him get his leave to remain in the UK but it will cost him money. He told Simon that he came to the UK some years back and when he came in, he came as a visitor. Having a visitor visa doesn't permit you to do any work in the UK and first time visitors are usually granted six months single entry visa from their home country. So he told Simon that, when he came to the UK he went to work illegally and he managed to raise some money and rent an apartment, then he had a Hungarian lady whom he paid about £5,000 to get married to. So that was how he got his right to be in the UK. Simon asked him what about the lady he got married to. He told him that she had gone back to her native Hungary. He told Simon that his application to the European Higher Court of Law will not succeed so therefore for him to be on the safer side, he should follow his advice and do what he tells him to do.

Simon was very desperate at that time. He didn't want to be deported to Nigeria with his present situation because it will be hell he may commit suicide. He then told him to give him a few days so he can contact those in charge of getting European Union ladies for marriage. He then told Simon that he will have to travel on his day off to Manchester to make an appointment with the Nigerians in charge running the sham marriage ring. Simon was very happy to hear this but he was not able to think about the consequences if he was caught. He just wanted to remain in the UK to continue to receive excellent treatment and a better life for he had no future in Nigeria.

Badejo left a few days after the day they spoke, to Manchester and he kept in touch with Simon throughout his time away. When he came back a few days after he told him they had helped him get a Spanish lady who has agreed to marry him, so he could get his leave to remain in the UK. He didn't tell his care coordinator or his psychiatrist because he warned Simon that what they are about to embark on is an illegal business so nobody should know about it if not they will go to jail or be deported to Nigeria but because he wanted to remain the UK, he kept it secret from his carers.

Badejo told Simon that it will cost him £6,000 for them to help him get his right to live in the UK. At that time he had £4,100 which he had saved, so he went to apply for a credit card with Lloyds TSB at that time and he borrowed £1,000 of credit. Badejo told Simon that he will have to pay £2,500 upfront for the process to begin and after the marriage with the Spanish lady then he can pay the balance of £3,500. Simon went to his bank that time and withdrew £2,500 cash from the counter and gave to him and he told Simon that he was travelling to Manchester to make the payment on his behalf. He left and came back a few days after and told Simon that the process had begun. Meanwhile Simon was still waiting for his application from the European Higher Court of Law. Simon's mental state started deteriorating further; he started hearing voices again and again and became suspicious of people. He would not eat nor do anything. He would stay indoors and not go for groups. His care coordinator would call him and try to find out what was wrong with him and ask why he wasn't in groups. She would sometimes come home to visit him. He used to tell her that he was frustrated and sick about his immigration worries which is having an impact on his health, even though he is trying to sort it out himself through an illegal means he was still worried and scared but he didn't tell her about trying to sort things out by illegal means. She would encourage him to come for the groups and booked to see him more frequently than before.

A few days after Simon heard a voice telling him that he will fail in his application so therefore he should go and hide all the money he has. Simon called Badejo that day and told him that he used to hear voices and one of the voices he just heard told him to hide all his money. So he told him that he should give him his account number so he can hide his money. He gave Simon his account number but the name on the account was Victor Michael. Simon asked him how come the name was different from his original Nigerian name, he told him that when he got married to the Hungarian lady that he changed his name at that time. So that was the name he bears. So Simon withdrew all the money from his account and from his credit card all in total was £2,600 cash which he went to deposit in Badejo's account. Simon never knew what he was doing at that time because he was so paranoid about the voices he heard. But that was the last time he ever saw Badejo again. Badejo disappeared with all his money which in total was £5,100. This had a very negative effect on Simon's health. His mental state fell further as a result of that. Badejo left his bags and belongings and never came back to collect them, till this day Simon don't know where Badejo could be found. Simon started losing concentration where he worked as a cleaner. He could not meet up to the standard of the job anymore. The teachers and head teacher in the school would complain to the agency that employed him. Simon was called up twice by his employer to tell him to improve in his job or else they would take him to another school. Simon started to emaciate because he could not eat properly and thinking about his condition. He was just looking for a way out of the situation. It was a very difficult time for him because he knew no one in the UK except his friends he met in the hospital. They get admitted in hospital sometimes because of relapse and he would visit them in hospital. They were his only family in the UK. He liked to go out and meet people sometimes but he got so scared if anyone got to know about his medical condition. He lives a one way life at the time. But deep within him, he knows he is a great person and has a nice personality but this is masked by his illness. His carers were doing a great job but he was still limited to some of the things other patients can access like welfare benefit and other things which other patients with the right documents would have. He was just a service user with no future for himself because of his immigration status. Getting treatment to Simon, at that time was just like pouring water into a basket and expecting the water would stay.

Simon resorted to online dating to save himself. He went on a dating website having a thought that he will find someone to marry or start a relationship with. This was in July 2009. A few days after he registered on that site and paid to become a member he met a lady called Jessica Ward who lives in Darlington in county Durham in the Northeast of England. They talked for almost a week online and she invited him to come to her house in Darlington.

At this time his mental state had deteriorated to the point that he started to hear voices and become suspicious of people and it became stronger than before. He lost appetite at this time and he always spent time on the internet. Anytime he started having early warning signs, he would usually lose appetite, lose weight, become suspicious of people, confused, hearing voices, having insomnia, getting personal messages either from the newspapers, radio or television and this signs becomes very strong if he stopped or continued not taking his medication or when alone. That night he was really restless because he couldn't sleep. He kept calling Jessica on the phone throughout that night. He felt like there were some unseen being in his flat trying to pass a message across to him and at the same time he was confused and couldn't control his thinking. The voices kept tormenting Simon and at a point it told him that he was going to die again and told him if he doesn't leave immediately with his belongings in the next one hour he will die. Simon became so scared and he quickly started packing up his clothes, shoes and other things he could pick up. At around 4am he quickly left his apartment with his belongings heading to Victoria Coach Station in London to buy a ticket to Darlington.

While he was in the Bus the voices kept tormenting him more and more repeating the things it's been saying to him. Simon's second episode was quite a bit different from his first but it was very similar because the voices kept saying the same things to him but the difference was that he became jealous about Jessica Ward and it was like the voice keep coming like a recording tape telling him things about her and trying to create anxiety in his head making him panic. Also his second episode was very strong, it was like a real voice not just an ordinary one it was like someone was actually talking to him using the microphone but he couldn't see them. It was very frightening and alarming. Simon would move from one seat to another seat in the Bus trying to avoid the voice. But it just seemed wherever he goes the voices follow him. Having a nap would have been better but he can't because he was so scared to do that and not just that the voices won't allow him and he haven't had his medication close to a year before he had his second episode. Simon's second episode is one he will never forget. At a point in time he replied to the voices verbally while in the Bus.

Simon arrived at Victoria Coach Station in London around 5am in the morning so had to wait till around 8am when the customer services opened for ticket sales. He quickly bought his ticket and waited for the Bus to leave around 9am. The Bus he took from the station was going to Newcastle and it passed through Darlington. Before he boarded the Bus he tried to call Jessica to tell her that he was on his way but she said he shouldn't come over again but he told her he had already bought the ticket then she dropped the phone. At this time he was disappointed but he said to himself he will still make his way to Darlington and try to ask her why she doesn't want him to come over. In the Bus he kept texting her telling her how far he was and updating her about his present destination. The Journey took seven hours he could remember from London Victoria Coach Station to Darlington. When he got to Darlington, he had spotted Jessica he quickly went to hug her and kissed her then he went to pick up his belongings from the Coach. She didn't give him a good look when she saw Simon with his belongings.

They got talking for a while and she took him to a local pub where she forced him to drink beer. He doesn't drink beer but that was the very first time he drank it. And he had much to drink that day because she kept urging him to drink and drink but because he just wanted to do what she said to please her. He kept drinking and drinking even though his body system would not allow him to. Simon got drunk that evening and she moved him to another pub where they had more to drink and eat. At the pub she was not happy to see him with his belongings so she was asking him why he had brought his belongings that they never agreed that he would move in with her. Simon told her "yes" that they didn't agree but he wants to start a new life with her and he was very scared to live in London alone. He told her that he was happy to be around her and he was safe. She look very baffled to hear him saying that to her. What you have read so far in this book and about to read further, are the best Simon can remember about what happened. This is his true story. Simon can promise anyone reading this book that the writings are events and happenings he has recorded as truthfully as he can remember as you can see these are not easy things to put in writing or talk about. Simon's illness sometimes makes him puzzled because he could remember most of his symptoms. It's very hard for someone with his condition to have every detail of events that took place when in a Schizophrenic episode. During this time he struggles with his thoughts and he felt safe when with someone he knows though the voices often come but less.

During Simon's time with Jessica, it appears as if the voices were reduced more than normal when he used to be alone. After the day she told him to go get some condoms in a shop and he went to buy about three packets and they went home. When they got home she told Simon to leave his belongings in the sitting room that she is not going to allow him live with her. Meanwhile when they were on their way to her house Simon kept telling her that he loves her and he wants them to have children together, she never gave him any response to all he said to her. Jessica was 38 at that time and she works for MIND helping the disabled.

Simon was 30 years and 4 months at the time. That night they both had sex. It was the very first time Simon made love to a woman in his life. After making love to her she asked Simon if he ejaculated and he said yes. She got so furious and told him that they agreed to use a condom but he didn't use it so she told him to leave her house and never return and that if he tries to come to find her, she said she will call the police and tell them that he was an illegal immigrant. As Simon was packing up all his belongings she told him that she had discussed with her best friend about him earlier and how he kept her up the previous night with phone calls and she was advised not to go ahead with the relationship that he just want to use her to get his legal right in the UK. Simon tried to convince her to let her know that he was genuine and not like any other person who would do such thing but she kept shouting and yelling at him threatening to call the police on him if he didn't leave. So Simon left her house in the middle of the night. It was around 2am in the morning that day.

Simon left Jessica's house and wandered in the street. As he walked alone in the middle of the night, shivering in the weather, he began to think about his life and ponder about the things happening to him. He was very scared and vulnerable at that time. He was thinking of going back to Jessica to beg her or speak to her friend who had advised her about him but he couldn't find his way back to her house because he had walked a very long distance from her house and made so many turns passing through so many streets. Then alas!! Came the voice again. Simon's biggest nightmare, it started to talk to him and repeated the same things he used to hear. It started telling him that he was a loser. It said he can't go back to London because he will die, then saying where will he live. It was like a mocking voice. Then he heard another voice saying to him to look for the nearest hospital to report that he needs help. This was the very first time he would hear another voice comforting him and given him an option to take unlike in his first episode he never had an optional voice except him trying to fight back the voice he hears.

Simon quickly changed the direction of his walk and started walking back the way he had come earlier. While he walked, he started looking for anyone around to ask where he can find the nearest hospital. What made him listen to the other voice remains a mystery to him. At this time he was very exhausted and thirsty. As he walked down the road he came across some teenagers who were having a nice time by the side of the road, he quickly walked down to them greeted them and asked them where he could find the nearest hospital. They were very nice and polite and they described to him how he could get to the nearest hospital by telling him to walk straight ahead and make a few turnings which he can't really remember the full description even now. From their look they felt pity and were wondering what was wrong with him. They asked him if he was alright and he replied yes and said thank you and left them. Simon had wanted to hang out with them but was just thinking they might not want to or maybe they were too young for him and he was just a stranger to them.

At this time Simon was so scared and wondering and asking himself if he was alright. The voice came back again telling him to remember the incident in the library when he assaulted a lady and telling him that he is in a big danger because he was where no one knows him and telling him that he had no escape. It even put impressions in his mind that his family in Nigeria are all dead and he is the last man standing and he was going to die like them. At this time he started running. He ran for about five minutes and stopped at a junction thinking the voice will go away. The voice came back again persecuting. Simon lost his direction to the hospital as described to him, then he was very confused and thinking he should be dead instead of passing through all these experiences.

Then Simon heard another voice again telling him to stop the nearest vehicle that come along the road he walked and asked for directions to the nearest hospital. As he walked along, there came a car he tried to wave it to stop but the driver didn't so he continued walking. Another car came along he did the same but it wouldn't stop. Simon came to another junction then contemplating which way to take whether right or left. He turned left and continued walking. He didn't know where he was going he was just wandering about the streets that night. Then another car came, he waved for it to stop and finally he got what he wanted, it stopped. Then he greeted the driver, he was an Asian probably an Indian or Pakistani descent and he asked him where the nearest hospital is. He asked Simon if he was sick, he told him that he is not sure but he would need to speak to a doctor to find out what was really wrong with him because he could hear voices. He was a very nice man he told him to get in the front seat and he will take him to the hospital.

Simon got in the front seat and he drove off. As he drove he felt drowsy. He asked him for his name and asked where he came from. He asked Simon if he lived around. He told him he was from London but found himself in the streets and he just wanted to speak to a doctor to report that there are some voices following him. He said alright. In no time they got to a hospital and he thanked him and told him to beware of the night, Simon didn't know why he said that to the young man probably because he was paranoid at the time. He told Simon goodbye and drove off.

Simon walked slowly into the entrance of the hospital and as he walked into the hospital it appears the voices were fighting within him, the first voice and the other voice. He approached the reception and asked to speak with a doctor on duty. They asked him his name he gave them his first name and he was asked his last name but he didn't tell them. The receptionist told him that without his full name and date of birth they can't confirm who he was and he can't see the doctor. They asked him where he was from he told them London. Then they ask where he lives. He told them he had nowhere to live but he just got kicked out by his girlfriend. They asked for his girlfriend's name and number so they could contact her. Simon gave them Jessica's number. So they phoned up Jessica and asked her if she knows anyone named Simon that he is in the hospital and that he was the one who gave them the number to call that she threw him out and stated he was her boyfriend. But Jessica denied ever knowing Simon saying she doesn't know anyone called Simon and she had never met him. Simon was unable earlier to tell his full name and date of birth to the receptionist because he was afraid to say his name because he was afraid of the voice he heard. The voice he heard was threatening and persecutory.

At that time he thought saying a different name would help him and also would give him a different personality which the voices he hears at that time will be afraid of. For example the name Andrews came to his head as a surname. He had thought that if he had said Simon Andrews that would have given him a different personality thereby scaring the voices from speaking to him. Simon had thought of Andrews at that time because Prince Andrew was one of the Royal family and no one really know much about him like other members of the Royal family. So he had thought if he had taken up Andrews as a surname then, it makes him a member of the Royal family therefore the voices would stop speaking to him because he will be seen as a Prince. Simon was so confused that the name he told the police officers during his first episode kept coming to his head but he could know at this time that his name was Simon. In his thought at that time he didn't see the receptionist as a doctor and never thought at that time that she was only trying to help him.

CHAPTER SIX
LIFE AFTER AND SECOND DISCHARGE

The receptionist took Simon to a room and told him to sit down and a doctor will be with him in few minutes. In that room he fell asleep and got a tap on his shoulder and when he woke up he saw two police officers in front of him smiling and said "hello" to him. At this time he was confused. Simon asked them if they have come to arrest him and what has he done. They kept smiling at him and trying to calm him down. They asked for his name he gave them his first name and they asked him for his date of birth he told them that he can't remember. Simon told them that he hears voices in his head and he was unable to control his thoughts. They asked him where he was from, he told them London. They asked him if he lives in London or Darlington. Simon said at the moment he have nowhere to live because his girlfriend threw him out of the house. They asked what her name was, he told them Jessica. Then they asked him where she lives he told them he really didn't know that he just found himself in the hospital. They asked him if he had any mental health history he told them NO!!! Simon said to them that he was fine but just wanted to speak to a doctor maybe the doctor can help or know how to reduce the voices he hears.

Then one of the officers left the room and left him with the other officer. At this time he was so tired, thirsty and confused. Simon was imagining how come the police officers are there in the hospital and why they are interrogating him. At the same time he felt settled a bit because in his head he was speaking to the voice in his mind saying that "The police are here so therefore he is safe and he will not die and he was telling the voice within him that the police will arrest it if they try to speak to him again" The other officer left with him in the room was a female and she was a blonde haired with blue eyes and was just smiling at him. Simon asked her what her name was and she told him Michelle and he said what a nice name. She told Simon that he will be fine and he should just relax. After this time he didn't hear any voice again. It was like the voices were scared to talk to him in presence of the police officer. Simon felt just like he was at home and the officers were assuring and calmed him down and always smiling at him. Before he knew it he fell asleep again and was woken up again by the male officer who left the room earlier. At this time he asked if Simon was alright and how he was feeling he told him that he was feeling well and much better and told them to please get him a place to stay because he can't continue to be on the streets. He told Simon that they are taking him to the police station to find out who he was first then they will sort out an accommodation for him.

When he got out of the hospital with the officers, it was dawn already and it was about 8am in the morning. All this took place around the end of July 2009. The officers took Simon into their car and drove him to Darlington Police Station. At the station they asked him his name again he only told them his first and asked to speak to a doctor. Then the officers started laughing and told him sure he will see a doctor but they need to know who he was first. Then they took him to a room, he had his finger prints taken and there it goes his full details appeared on the screen. Then they asked him if he was the person whose name just appeared on the screen? He told them NO!!! It's not me. Then they burst into laughter again. At this time they took him to another room and told him to have a rest while they try to sort an accommodation for him. Simon was very happy to hear that an accommodation will be sorted. In the room he fell asleep again and the officers would come from time to time to wake him up and ask if he was alright. The officers instructed him not to leave the police station and if he needs anything he should let them know.

At a time he became impatient and wanted to go out to look at the surroundings. It just felt like he found himself a new home. But he kept thinking about Jessica and wanted to see her again. Simon walked out of the police station and had a short stroll for about a few yards from the station and the environment was so beautiful. There was a Church of England just opposite the police station. Simon didn't want to go too far because he have been instructed not to leave the station so he walked back and pressed on the buzzer and someone picked up and it sounded like Jessica, he quickly asked if it was Jessica, the person asked who Simon was. Simon told the lady on the phone that he was brought to the station by two police officers and they were trying to sort out an accommodation for him, so he just went for a walk, and he was allowed in. Simon was really hallucinating at that time thinking that it was Jessica because she was in his mind throughout that time.

The officers came back to him and were asking him if he had an application with the Home Office which was in court at that moment he told them yes. Then they told him that they have got no accommodation for him and they will need to report him to the Home Office, Simon replied to them that if they can't provide him with an accommodation then he will have to go live with the Home Office because he won't go anywhere. Then they smiled at him and then asked him his name again he told them his first name and said Andrews as his surname. Then they said wow!!! You have now beginning to remember your surname that's excellent!!! But it is different from the one in the database how come? Simon told them that there must have been a mistake somewhere. They started smiling at him again and said he can choose whatever name he wished to tell them but they will have to follow what name they see on the database. Simon told them to change his surname on the database that he didn't want that name that he wanted Andrews as his surname. Then they laughed and said they can't change it that the name has to stay on the system like that but if he had to change it, then he can do that himself later when he is alright.

Simon told them that he was alright he just needed to speak to a doctor to find out about some of the things happening to him because he hears voices. They told Simon he will soon see a doctor. Then they asked him if he could remember his date of birth he told them no. They smiled at him again and said alright they got an accommodation for him but it's a mental health hospital which he would need to go and stay. They asked him if he have ever been to a mental health hospital before he told them he was not sure. At this time he was very tired and just wanted to sleep and at the same time want to talk to Jessica. Talking to the officers really relieved Simon of the stress he was going through at that time and it appears the voices died down a bit during this time.

So Simon was taken to the police car and driven to a psychiatry hospital in Darlington. The police officers told him "this is your new home". They lead him through the entrance and a psychiatry nurse came and ushered him in and the police officers stayed with him for a while. He thanked the officers and told them he would like to see them some other time and they smiled at him and drove off. While in the hospital, the psychiatry nurse asked Simon if he knew where he was. He replied to her that he was in the hospital and she asked him what kind of hospital he think he was in. Simon told her that he doesn't know. Then she told him that he was in a mental health hospital. Simon was made to sit down for a while in a place that looked like a canteen in the hospital. The nurse was very friendly and kept reassuring him that he will be fine. All he just wanted to do that time was to have somewhere to sleep. They sat down for a while the nurse was talking to him and she asked him if he wanted anything to drink. Simon told her yes he would like a glass of water. She provided him with water and smiled at him. Simon was relieved for a while when he was in the hospital but he kept thinking in his mind if he was really sick and where he would go from the hospital after discharge. He began to worry and thinking all sorts running through his head. He started becoming paranoid again and thinking maybe it's a plot by the police officers to leave him in hospital with the nurses to kill him in secret since no one knows where he was. He became very fearful and wondering what's going to happen to him.

What the entire message the nurse was telling him at that time began to seem like a plot, he became very suspicious and thinking whether the water she gave him was not poisoned. He started thinking about his family in Nigeria, trying to ponder what the voices had told him earlier that his family are all dead. Simon's illness makes him out of touch with reality sometimes even though he gets assurance from people around. He often tends to believe the voices and see it as reality. Simon is telling you this story how he felt at that time so you reading this book will understand the true mind of a Paranoid Schizophrenic individual, how they think, perceive and see things when they show their strong symptoms in other words when they are sick.

It's a very hard experience to explain. Simon would imagine you being in his thoughts all that time, to know exactly how to explain the symptoms very well. Most people need to be aware of mental illness in society and know how to relate with mentally ill people and the type of care they need. He has had excellent treatment so far compared to if he was in Nigeria. He had stopped taking his medication on the second occasion when he fell ill, but it took a while before he started experiencing any symptoms about close to nine months. This Simon thinks is probably due to the psychosocial activity he was involved in and other treatment apart from the medication. If he had stayed on his medication throughout plus other treatment he wouldn't have had a relapse the second time. Also the situation around Simon about his immigration status contributed 90% to his breakdown.

The nurse took him in and introduced him to other staff in the ward and other patients as well and told him he can make a coffee or tea to drink and showed him how to do that. He was placed in an acute ward. This ward is for patients whose illness is not so severe like others. While in the Hospital he began to think about Jessica and wouldn't talk to anyone. Then he heard the voice again but this time it was soft telling him that Jessica has been looking for him. He started hallucinating again. He went to the staff and told them that he wanted to go and see Jessica. They asked him who Jessica was he told them she was the woman he met on a dating site a few weeks ago and he came to Darlington to see her. They told him that he can't see her and tried to calm him and talk to him. But he got very angry while the staff talked to him, he ran to the entrance where the ward door was and gave it a very hard kick!!! The door came widely open and he ran out of the ward, trying to escape out of the hospital to go and find Jessica. Before he knew it, a very loud alarm started sounding and it brought the attention of other staff members in the hospital and they all chased Simon and caught up with him. They took him back to the hospital and quickly injected him and he didn't know anything that happened after then. When he woke up he found himself in a different ward. This time they now put him in the severe ward. This is the ward for people who are more violent or whose psychiatry illness is very serious.

Simon woke up with a strong weakness, looked around it was very dark in the room he was at that time. He stood up from his bed got his feet on the floor trying to find the switch but he could see partially because of the reflection of the lights from the corridor. The door to his room had glass in through which you can see the corridor and anyone outside can see through. In no time he found the switch and switched on the light in the room he was in. OH!!! What a day that was for him. He was still scared at that time. He slowly walked out of his room, looked round the corridor and went back to his room. Simon stayed in the room for a while peeping through the window and trying to observe the environment.

Then suddenly a nurse came to do the normal routine check and saw him up. “Hello Simon” he said and “How are you”? Simon replied “I am fine. He told Simon they will soon have dinner so he should get ready to join other patients. He then said ok. He walked out of his room and started wondering along the corridor, walking to and fro. The other staffs noticed him and one of them came to him and asked him if he would like to have a chat before dinner. He said he was alright but he would like to speak with the consultant of the ward and he wants to see his care coordinator, Christine Baker. He told him that he will see the consultant on the day of the ward round and as regards to his care coordinator he will be taken back to London very soon to be admitted in a hospital where he originally lives then he can see his care coordinator. Then he asked him if there is any more he had to say, Simon told him no that he was fine.

Simon had dinner that evening and the staffs were very friendly and helpful towards him. Before the day of the ward round, he was in his room lying down on his bed covered with the duvet. He had a knock on the door and it was one of the nurses. He told him that a doctor wants to speak with him. Simon got up and went with him and he was made to sit down near the dining hall, waiting for few minutes before he was called into a room. The doctor was a Ugandan. He was ushered into the room and he asked him his name. He told him Simon Andrews. He said but that's not the name he's got in his record. He then told Simon that his care coordinator has been very worried about him because they have been looking for him. He told him that they will have to send him back to London where he will be admitted to a hospital close to his house because that's where his care is located. Simon told him "No he can't go back to London that he will die." He told him that they should look for a council accommodation for him in Darlington. He told Simon that he is not eligible for a council accommodation because he has no legal status in the UK. He then asked him what medication he was on, Simon replied Risperidone and he asked how many milligrams. He told him he can't remember. He asked him how long ago he had taken his medication, he told him a very long time ago around September 2008.

When he was talking to Simon, one of the ward nurses was with him looking at him and smiling and as he asked him questions he was writing on a file. At the end of the discussion, he told Simon that they had received a report from his carer in London and he will be due to see the ward consultant before he will be taken to London.

Simon waited patiently for the day of the ward round, on that day it was a Friday and he was made to see the consultant. He was ushered in on that day with a staff nurse already in position, sitting opposite the consultant. He walked in and he was greeted by the doctor. He asked him his name he told him Simon Andrews, he said no your name is Simon Algood he said no I don't want that surname. He asked him why. Simon told him that if he accepted that name then he will continue to hear voices and have a different personality. He told him he was scared of the voices he hears and it's because of the name he bears. He asked him why he picked up the name Simon Andrews. He explained to him that one of the Royal family member's names is Prince Andrew and no one hears about him like Prince Philip, Harry, Charles or William so therefore he is taking up the name Andrews so that the voices he hears will be scared of him because they will see him as a Prince. Then Simon asked him if he believe in GOD or if GOD exists? He replied to him that he is not going to discuss anything about faith with him. He then asked him how long he had been in Darlington. He told him he can't remember. He asked him what brought him to Darlington. Simon told him that he came to see his girlfriend and he was scared of going back to London. He asked him why he was scared to go back. He told him the voices warned him not to go back there. He asked him are the voices speaking to him now as he speaks to him. Simon replied they always speak with him but not at the moment because it's faint but he could still hear them. He asked him why he kept disturbing the lady he came to see in Darlington, with calls the other night. Simon shouted suddenly at the top of his voice saying "I came to take back what belongs to me", then he shook his hands and said that's the end of his meeting with him and he said they will see again at their next ward round.

Simon left his presence and went into his room. At that time he felt a little headache and he went to sleep. Simon never had time to see the doctor again because he was driven by two staff nurses in the car back to London. During the journey, he slept all through and when he woke up he found himself in London. He was woken up by the nurses and they told him that he was now in Highgate Hospital in Archway, North London. He was taken to a ward. The nurses were very friendly and professional. One of the nurses took him to his room and showed him how to use the shower and said if he had any problem he should feel free to let the nurses know then they left him in the room. Simon looked outside the window where his room was, there was a fence and over the fence was a cemetery. Quickly he heard the voices again saying to him “welcome back”. He quickly left the room and went to the nurses and told them he wanted another room. They asked him why. He told them that he can hear spirits from the cemetery. They told him that he will be fine that there are no spirits in his room and the cemetery has been there for a very long time and no spirit has ever spoken to any patient who has been in the room before him so he should keep calm. They told Simon they had informed his care coordinator that he was now in the hospital and that he has been brought back to London so he will be seeing her in few days plus he will be seeing the ward doctor at the ward round very soon. Then they suggested to him that he should not look through the window and he should always have the curtains closed so he doesn’t hear voices from or look at the cemetery. That relieved him a bit.

On the day of the ward round, his care coordinator came to see him and she asked him why he stopped taking his medication and kept it secret. He apologised and told her he was frustrated about his immigration situation and that he has a huge debt and had been thinking of paying it back. She asked him how he got himself into debt and how much was it. Simon told her that he borrowed money from the bank. He didn’t know what will happen if he had told her what he used the money for and how he was scammed. She asked him how long before that time he had stopped taking his medication. He told her he had stopped taking it since September the previous year.

Simon told her to please help him get in touch with Jessica. Then she told him that he should leave the woman in peace that he had lost her already, that he would have to start a new life afresh.

She then told him that she will be leaving the service on a year training so she will have to transfer his care to another psychiatry nurse but he will still be under her care until she leaves. She told him that she has to trust him because he didn't tell her the truth when he stopped taking his medication. Then she said he will be more closely monitored than before and ensure he takes his medication. Then she told Simon he will be seen in few minutes by the ward doctor, Dr Gerrard. In about ten minutes he was called into a room by one of the ward nurses on duty. In the room was seated his care coordinator, the ward doctor, two other doctors and a ward nurse. The ward doctor greeted him and told him to have a seat. Simon was seated facing the other mental health professionals. She asked him why he stopped taking his medication and kept it secret from his care coordinator. Simon apologised to her and to his care coordinator that it will never happen again. Then he asked her where will he go when discharged from hospital, she told him that he will go back to where he used to live provided by the no recourse to public funds team because his service with them still runs until the following year before they will stop any support and transfer him to a local GP. Then she said he should not worry about his accommodation he should just focus on his health and if he need any help the nurses are there for him to help out.

She asked him about his mood and about the voices he hears. Simon told her the voices are beginning to disappear and he was due for discharge. She said no he was not due for discharge she is the psychiatric doctor and will know when and decide the time when he will leave hospital. There was another doctor who was observing Simon as he spoke and was typing on the computer and smiling to him on occasion. At that time he felt a bit better because the voices he heard had started to disappear gradually. That's the effect of his medication; as soon as he resumes taking it, in a few days or weeks he begins to feel different. The medication really helps in killing the voices it's like magic.

Simon's care coordinator really helped him in encouraging him telling him that he shouldn't worry that his appeal in the European court will come out successful so he should not bother about it. The mental health professionals were his family at that time. He had another ward round in the hospital. This time he was well enough to be discharged and was discharged in August 2009. He didn't spend too much time in hospital during his second episode. He left the hospital by himself and went home. But meanwhile he had already moved from Islington to Enfield borough.

CHAPTER SEVEN
MY LIFE AS A PSYCHIATRY PATIENT

When Simon got home he saw a letter in his flat and it was from his employer telling him to report to the office or he will lose his job. On the day he got home, the door was widely open, not locked and the flat was scattered. He quickly recollected what had happened to him when the voices were threatening him to leave and how he left in haste. Simon cried and had pity for himself but comforted himself and began rearranging his flat again and cleaning everywhere.

On that same day he went to his employer and they told him that it has been over a month since he left his job without informing them. They said they tried to call his number but it was switched off so they were wondering what had happened to him. Simon had never missed work since he started working with them they said. Then they said he should explain himself why did he really decide to report himself if it was because of the letter they sent him. He told them he was very sorry that he had not been at work for close to a month never knew it was that long but he pleaded with them to allow him to continue with the job and he told them he was admitted in psychiatry hospital because he had a relapse and didn't know what he was doing. Simon told them that he just got discharged. So he was asked to provide his discharge certificate from the hospital he was admitted and the dates he went into hospital and when he left, before they will continue to employ him. Simon left his employer's office that day and the next day he went to get his discharge certificate from the patient's affairs and took it to his employer. Simon was very lucky and he was allowed to continue to work.

Simon started a new life again, living on his own, attending groups when necessary, visiting his two friends and meeting up with his care coordinator but he was still not thinking he was safe because he didn't know what the outcome of his appeal would be at that time. He spoke to his family back in Nigeria at that time and he did send money to them when necessary but never told them all he had gone through. He kept it secret from them. Simon only told them he was admitted to hospital but didn't tell them the nature of his sickness. He kept taking his medication and remained compliant.

Everything started going on well with him again. At that time he was saving to pay off his credit card debt and the loan he took out which went through the drain through scam. Simon was able to save until around end of 2009 and he cleared off the credit card debt and was very happy and he was left with the loan which he was paying off gradually.

But meanwhile before this time, he went back to the dating website where he met Jessica and tried to search for a lady. He did that because he was not sure of his appeal and the immigration solicitor has told him earlier that he have a 50 50 chance of success and he had been advised by his friends to have a backup in case his appeal don't come out successful. He met a lovely lady from the site who happened to come from one of the European Union countries. They have met twice since the past four years she had come to visit the UK and they met and she has been a very good friend to Simon and like a mother to him. Her name was Ellen Roberto. Ellen has helped Simon in several ways in aspects of moral support, giving him money, and helping him with shopping. Some of the things in his flat today were bought by her. He thanked GOD for ever knowing her and they are best friends forever.

He met several other ladies during this time but they often disappear when they know the country he comes from. Not only that a majority of them wouldn't like to have anything to do with him. The moment they discover he does not have a legal status at that time. This resulted in his isolation and he wouldn't want to interact with any lady. Simon also developed fear and became very timid in approaching any lady. He was still strong and continued living his normal life. Sometimes he did hang out with his friends Friday and Grace and they would go out for shopping together, go to a restaurant or just stay at home entertaining each other. They were his family at that time and encouraged and gave him moral support. They encouraged each other to continue with their medication even though they themselves sometimes didn't take the medication and then falling sick. .He lived a lonely life and wouldn't talk to anyone except the people he meet during the groups organised by the mental health workers. He got frustrated in his life because he couldn't meet anyone to have a serious and genuine relationship with.

One day he went to visit one of his friends Grace and she told him she would like them to go out to a restaurant to eat because she wants to give him a treat. So she asked him where is the best place to go out to enjoy good Nigerian food. Simon told her there was one he knows in Woolwich in southeast London and it's called "Tasty". So she said they should go there. They took the bus from where she lives around Mornington Crescent Station to Euston Station and took a train to London Bridge and then from there to Woolwich Arsenal Station. The restaurant was just a few minutes' walk from the station. When they got to the restaurant, they ordered food and as they enjoyed their food with a malt drink, Simon received a phone call and when he looked at it, it was his immigration solicitor. My goodness!!! His heart began to beat faster than normal. He was just looking at the phone ringing then, Grace asked him "why don't you want to pick your call and who was that"? Before she could finish he pressed on the answer button and said "Hello". The person on the other end said this is Sheena Jacob "can I speak to Mr Simon Algood please"? He replied "speaking".

She then broke the bad news to him she said the European High Court of Law upheld the decision which means that is the end of any appeal right he have and said there is nothing more she could do. She told him she will send the decision notice to him and his file will be closed. She told him that he can choose to leave the UK and go back to Nigeria voluntarily or continue to live in the UK without a legal status for the next fourteen years and then apply for amnesty thereafter, but he should be warned if he got involved with the police or any immigration officials in any case or circumstance then he could be deported she said. Then she said she is very sorry about the decision and she dropped the phone. At that moment he paused for few moments staring at his phone and began thinking of what next to do. Grace was very anxious and she asked him what the matter was. Simon couldn't look at her to explain anything. He felt like crying.

From that moment Simon became a confirmed illegal immigrant in the UK. He and Grace started staring at each other then she asked him if he was alright. He told her it was his immigration solicitor who just called and she asked him ""so"".... Then he said he lost his final appeal which means he is an illegal immigrant. At that time they couldn't eat their food anymore. This was around November 2009. Grace felt like crying on that day. She sees Simon as her younger brother and seeing things like that happen to him really touched her. She tried to encourage him and told him that he just needed to find someone to be in a relationship with, someone who will understand his situation.

That was the beginning of another nightmare in Simon's life. He started thinking how he will get out of his current situation, with immigration rules in the UK beginning to tighten up every year. How will he find a genuine person? So many things started running through his mind. He had thought that leaving the UK entirely was an option. He could maybe go to another European country but how can he cross the borders of the UK without a valid visa? Besides he has no passport, he had thrown it away when he was sick during his first episode. He started thinking about his life because at that time he has no option at all. He had been frustrated by ladies who don't want to have anything to do with him because of his country of origin or because of his legal status. But Grace started encouraging him and told him to be patient and told him that the right person will come his way at the right time saying he should not give up hope. They left the restaurant that day in a gloomy countenance and she told him these are hard times for him and he should stay in touch with his care coordinator and keep taking his medication. She told him something will happen but it might not be immediately. Simon followed her back home and stayed with her for a while before he left.

When Simon got home, he was very worried and scared that the immigration officers will come knocking at his door. He got in touch with his family in Nigeria to explain to them his condition concerning his immigration status in the UK but didn't tell them he was receiving treatment or about his mental health. Then he called his father to know if he has got any distant relative living in London or anywhere in the UK whom he could go and live with and leave his present accommodation. He told Simon he doesn't have any contact with his family living in the UK but he knows he's got some family members. He told him to help him find out as soon as possible because he doesn't want to be deported. In a few days Simon's father phoned him and gave him a number to call, telling him the number belongs to one of his nephews who once lived with him when Simon was still a baby. He told him he was the person who helped him to get to the UK in the early 80s. So therefore he should call him that they have already spoken on the phone few days earlier. He quickly called the number in no time. He picked up his call, his name was Tejiri. Simon asked to speak to Tejiri and he introduced himself. He was not speaking to him in a friendly manner at that time. So he asked Simon "what can I do for you" Simon explain to him he had just lost his appeal to the European High Court of Law to see if he could assist him to get a new immigration solicitor to make a fresh application. He told him to come see him at his store the next day and he gave him his store address at Deptford High Street in southeast London. Simon called Grace and Friday and he told them that he had been able to locate one of his relatives in London.

The next day he went to see him and he told him that he should not be afraid that the Home Office will never come to find him that he should be at peace. Simon told him about his medical condition and his hospital admissions. He asked him if he had gotten better and Simon told him yes. He said on his immigration issue there is nothing he could do to help him with that but what he can do for him is to help him get a job with one of his friends who works in a club. He asked him if he had ever worked in a club before and if he can do the job. Simon told him he can do any job and he is not job shy.

Meanwhile at that time he work part time as a cleaner in the mornings, so getting another part time job will help him pay off his debt quickly. He told him about how he was scammed he was very sorry to hear that. He told Simon to be strong and advised him to always keep in touch; he said he needs to know him better. Simon kept going to visit his Uncle, Tejiri from time to time sometimes he would call him.

In 2010 around January Simon received a phone call by one of his uncle's friends his name was Isaac. He told him that he was his uncle's friend and that he gave him his number. He asked Simon if he was available to work at the weekend. He explained the nature of the job to him. The job was working as a washroom attendant in a club. The job involved staying in a washroom where you display all sorts of aftershaves, sweets, chewing gum with a tiny tray where people can leave you with money after using aftershaves or products you have displayed. It also involved soliciting for money and talking to people who have come to use the toilet. That was the job he got at that time in the club and it was very rewarding because you don't have to present any documents and it was tax free. But there was a policy that the men would always pay the contractor at the end of the day and it could be anything that ranged from £10 to £20 depending on how busy the club was that day. The job really helped Simon that time because he combined his morning cleaning job with the weekend job. Simon was able to have some savings at that time.

CHAPTER EIGHT
SECOND RELATIONSHIP

In February 2010, just before valentine day Simon registered to use another dating website and he met a lady called Julia King. They chatted for the first time and she seemed very friendly. They chatted again the second time and he asked her how long she has been on the site and if she had got kids. Julia was 32 years and 5 months when Simon met her at that time. Simon was 31 years and 11 months at the time. They met again the third time and they met again the fourth time and they became very close friends. Then she gave him her phone number. Simon and Julia chatted every day and most times they would make an appointment to meet up to chat online. Julia had three kids at the time. Simon's interest for Julia began to grow and she started developing strong feelings for him. About four months after they had been chatting online they decided to meet up in person. Although Julia had already told him that she was seeing a guy called Peter but she said their relationship was not a serious one that they were just friends.

Julia lived outside London at the time. She was living in Gillingham in Kent. From London to Gillingham was about one hour plus by train. Simon travelled one Saturday to visit Julia. He got to Gillingham Station but meanwhile she had advised him to come out of the station and wait for a while that she will be with him in a few minutes. Simon waited for about ten minutes and he got a text telling him to walk to an orange coloured golf car. He looked round and saw a golf car, parked in front of the station and behold was Julia at the passenger's seat waving for him to come over. He walked to the car and they hugged each other and she lifted the seat for him to go to the back seat. She introduced him to her friend Deborah who was driving the car and also introduced him to her daughter Samantha who was the last of her three kids.

Deborah drove to Julia mum's house to drop them there. Julia had already told Simon earlier that she was going to see her mum to prepare her medication and asked if it's ok with him to go with her. He had agreed before then. Deborah dropped them off at Julia's mum and drove off. Simon, Julia and her baby daughter Samantha walked into a cottage house and she introduced him to her mother as her new friend. Simon felt very welcome. She served him with a soft drink and they got talking for a while. They spent some time there about three hours. Simon was busy watching TV and playing with the cat. Simon loved the cat a lot. After a while they got prepared to leave and Julia's mum who told Simon she would like to see him again and called him a gentleman. They left and headed to Julia's house. They took the public transport; it took about 35 minutes to get to Julia's house from her mum's.

When they got to her house she introduced him to her son Michael who had been on the computer playing a game. She asked Simon if he wanted anything to drink he told her yes just a glass of water. She provided him with water and cooked lunch for the household. He was there that day for a long period of time and he watched a football match in her house. She was very friendly and her son Michael was very funny because they got talking. After eating lunch he told her he would like to leave and she called her friend Deborah to come and drop him off at the station where he would get a train back to London. Deborah lived with her partner at that time just right at the back of where Julia lives. In a few minutes she drove and waited outside, Simon and Julia came out of the house and entered the car and told the kids goodbye. Along the way Deborah told Simon that she would like to meet him again though they didn't have time to sit and talk because she was busy at her own house.

She told Simon that she will be organising a picnic in a few weeks from that time and would like to invite him. Simon was very happy to hear this. At this time it just seemed like every worry he had had disappeared he didn't think of any immigration status or his mental health issues. It just seemed like everything had started to fall into place for him. At that time he was thinking of the possibility of himself and Julia dating in the future. They got to Gillingham Station and she pulled up at the car park, gave him a hug and a soft kiss on his cheek and Julia did the same to him and he came out of the car and waved to them and left.

Simon took the train from there and went home to prepare for his work at the club. He worked at the club every weekend and realised some money which he used to support himself and from time to time he would send money to his younger siblings. During this time he was taking his medication and seeing his care coordinator as usual so he didn't have any relapse. He was really doing well at this time. Simon and Julia continued chatting online on msn, Facebook and they could text each other often several times in a day. Their closeness became even stronger. Simon went to visit Julia one weekend and she told him that she is single again because the guy she was seeing, Peter had told her that he is not interested in a serious relationship with her, that he just wanted both of them to be casual friends. She told Simon she was not too bothered about it because their relationship was nothing serious in the first place.

At this time Simon didn't tell Julia about his immigration status in the UK or his mental health issues. They were just friends at that time and they kept the communication between them open. A few weeks after that time, Simon went to Gillingham to attend a picnic organised by Deborah and Collins. At that time Collins was Deborah's fiancé at that time. They went to a Park and played football and had a wonderful time at the time. At the Park Simon started telling Julia about his family background and he told her about his immigration status in the UK. She encouraged him and hoped that it would get sorted so he can move on with his life. After the picnic, they went to Deborah and Collins's house and watched football and played games. It was really fun that day and it was one of the days in Simon's life he would live to remember. Simon and Julia started having increased feelings for each other but no one could come out first to say it. Many times when he visited her he would want to break the ice but he would always lose courage and postpone it until another day. Sometimes she would text him that she misses him and asked when he was coming to visit her and the kids again and also saying that her friend Deborah and her mother always ask after him.

Simon became very happy about his relationship with Julia and he told his friends Grace and Friday about her and they told him to be patient with her and take things as it comes and said they should try to develop trust between each other. They were very happy for Simon to hear that he was doing very well. Meanwhile during this time Julia's mother has been asking her if they were already dating even Deborah and Collins was expecting them to start a relationship and every time Simon came to visit Julia and he left, Deborah would ask her what they discussed and she would be asking her when he was going to break the ice. Sometimes she encouraged Julia to say it first but she always replied that she is scared to say it first just in case he was not interested in a relationship with her. One Saturday in August 2010, Simon went to visit Julia and they had a good time together. They went to have a Chinese buffet meal together with her baby daughter Samantha and went to relax in a park. Gillingham is a nice place and very quiet and beautiful.

After the day he got prepared to leave and she followed him to the train station. On the way there he had it in his heart to break the ice that day. And at the Station he looked into her eyes, held her hands and told her that he has been in love with her for a long time but didn't know how to say it and he asked her if she would be his girlfriend. She gave him a big grin, looked to the floor, paused awhile looked to her side and finally she looked at him and said "YES". They then hugged each other and kissed. That was the very first time he kissed Julia and had a strong hug from her. He was very happy that day and so was she. He told her he will be coming to visit her and the kids the next weekend and told her to say "Hello" to her mum and her friend and he left. That day was like a dream come true. The next step he was thinking was to take it from there and his priority was to get engaged too Julia. She was a very lovely lady and since they love each other, then what stops them from getting married. She went home and the first person she called was her friend Deborah and she told her that finally Simon asked her out. They were so happy and her mother was very pleased to hear about it as well.

Simon and Julia became so much involved with each other and they could text each other more than a hundred times a day. He told her about his mental health issues at this time and she promised to support him in every way. A week after the day he asked her out, Saturday 4th September, he went to visit Julia and her friend Deborah came to pick him up at Gillingham Station and she congratulated them and said she was very pleased to hear that finally that they have both started a relationship and she shook his hands and told him that she will give them the necessary support to see them both happy. She drove them in her car to Julia's mother and her mother was very happy and pleased to see Simon and she said well done and hoped for a happy life together.

After spending time with her mother they left and Deborah drove Simon and Julia to her house and she left them to spend time together. Simon had never spent time alone with Julia before without the kids around. That day they made love. The second time he would ever have sex with a woman. It was passionate love making and at the end he could see the smiles in her face and she was a bit shy to look at him after then. He had gone to see Julia with some condoms but she had told him they would not need it because they should work towards having a baby. She had told him that she wants to give him a baby since he has never had a child in his life before.

After their love making they put on their clothes and within a short time Deborah came knocking with Samantha and they just said to each other that was right on time and they laughed between each other. Julia went to open the door for Deborah and Samantha and they came in and she asked them how their time was together. They smiled and said it was fine. They all stayed for a brief period chatting to each other and then he prepared to leave for home. Deborah took Simon in her car as usual and dropped him off at the train station. So he left that day.

Before Christmas of 2010, Simon got engaged too Julia and got her a ring which he got from an Argos store. Simon became involved with Julia's family because she introduced him to every member of her family. Simon always went to spend the weekend with her from Friday to Sunday and he would return back to London. During the time they were dating they never missed anytime without love making. Most times they would have sex up to four times a day. There was a day one of Julia's eldest kids Michael, asked them if they based their relationship just on sex alone because most times they had sex they could hear them from their room. Sometimes they mimic their moaning sounds during love making or would scream from their rooms and say "Please keep the noise down we have to sleep". They often got embarrassed by the kids knowing they were making love but that doesn't still stop them from making love when they had to. Sometimes they tried to wait until the kids were in bed before they make love, but sex was just something they enjoyed every day when Simon was around at the weekend.

Sometimes Julia would visit him in London when the kids were in school and she would go back just before the kids finished from school. Simon lived a very healthy lifestyle at that time. He was very happy and Julia always encouraged him to take his medication whenever he felt like stopping since he was doing really well. Simon and Julia started attending the Church of England together so they could get married. Simon got engaged to Julia in the presence of her mother when he bought her a ring. She was so happy and that was the beginning of a new life for them from that moment. Simon and Julia agreed to get married to each other on St Valentine's Day the next year which was in 2011. They were making plans towards this date.

A few days after they agreed to get married, Simon went to visit Julia and she told him that she had got something bothering her and told him that they should postpone their wedding until Sunday 12th February 2012 because it was too soon and they need to prepare very well in terms of arrangements and getting money to organise a wedding. She cited and gave reasons that they wouldn't have saved enough till the next year but if they could have it the following year then it would give them enough time and more money to have a successful wedding. Simon asked her whether it's not for any other reason she has changed the date. She told Simon "NO" it's just for that reason alone. She told him that she understands what his fears are but he should rest assured that nothing will happen before then and they will definitely get married at the right time. She told Simon that he was safe and he should not think of anything negative. She said he had always been a very good and gentle person and he got around with his own business so he should be fine.

She started crying and told him that she didn't want to lose him just because of this reason. Simon helped her wipe her tears and he told her that he had heard her and she should stop crying that she will never lose him. Simon told her that he was ready to wait till the year after the following year and he welcomed the idea. Then they made long passionate love again after talking. They went to see the Vicar of the church they attended and they told him about their intentions of getting married he took their details and recorded everything and put it in a file. He told them that they should continue attending the service and when it's close to the time they were to get married he will call them together to have a practice.

During this period he never showed any sign of mental illness and he was taking his medication as usual and doing relatively well. He became loved by the kids and sometimes he would tell Jokes with the eldest Michael. Simon and the Julia's youngest kid Samantha was born in the same month. On her birthday he bought her a scooter from the Argos store which she enjoyed riding on anytime they were out for a walk. Simon bought the eldest son Michael a dumbbell weight set for his own birthday when it came. And he gave her daughter Chelsea £30 for her birthday which was in January at that time because she said she didn't want a present but would prefer money. Simon fell in love with Julia every day that passed by and they maintained a very healthy relationship during the course of time. They exchanged their passwords on their Facebook account between each other at this time.

At a point in time Simon suggested to her that he could move in with her because they always missed each other during the week and only saw each other at weekends and the weekends went so fast. Sometimes at weekends he could only see her on a Saturday and wouldn't sleep over because of his commitment with his job at the club. Meanwhile in November 2010, Simon was able to pay off the rest of the loan he took out with Lloyds TSB Bank because he saved enough from the two jobs he was doing at that time. He was so happy at this time because this gave him extra comfort.

Julia told Simon that he couldn't move in with her because she was afraid of her neighbours or people around watching who might go to report to the council or benefit office that she's got a partner living with her. Julia was not working at that time and she had not worked for a period of six years up till that time. She then told Simon the story of her younger child, Samantha's father, that when they were dating someone went to report to the council that she's had a partner living with her which she hadn't declared to the council.

She told him that although she missed him during the week and wished that they were living together. She said the kids missed him too and are worried about her state during the week because during the week she was not a happy mother because she was alone with the kids except during the weekend when he is around. It's been difficult for her how she cope during the week she told Simon. At that time it was not easy for Simon as well because he had wanted to be with her all the time. They had no hitch in their relationship at this time but the problem of not seeing each other every day became a very big issue. Simon became more involved with her family and every weekend he would go to visit his fiancée they would go to see her mother and sometimes on occasion they would go to see one of her elder sisters Rebecca who was married at that time to his namesake Simon. Simon and he were good mates and they got along because they both liked football. He supports Arsenal while Simon was a Manchester United fan.

One day Simon, Julia's in-law held a birthday party and he was invited along with other members of Julia's family and some friends were present. That night Julia got drunk and he had to guide her home that evening but they still made love that night. Love making was a big part of their relationship and they never stopped making love when they were together. They would always make love every now and then and sometimes they would tell the kids to excuse them for some time. That time they were planning towards having kids together.

Simon lost his job at the club in November 2010 because he had fallout with the contractor concerning the issues of money and payment. So he was left with his cleaning job, but meanwhile because he was a very hardworking person and always punctual and had a good attendance record he was given extra hours to work in the evening in another school by the same cleaning agency. So he had a full time job at that time.

At this time he was living in the UK illegally but he had no contact with the police or the Home Office. His visa had expired two years before this time and his employers didn't check records or make any updates to his file so he continued working illegally in the UK at that time. His hope was waiting till February 2012 when he will be legally married to his fiancée Julia before he could renew his documents. He had a friend at that time whom he work with in the same company and they were very close at that time, he was advising him to save enough money that he will introduce him to his brother who was into sham weddings in the UK. They will get him someone to marry whom he will pay and then he can continue with his relationship with Julia at the same time. He advised Simon that he can't tell what might happen in the long run, so to be on the safer side he should get his right to remain in the UK on time instead of waiting till 2012. He told Simon success stories about the people who had done it through his brother and many of them now have legal rights to remain in the UK. He warned Simon so many times and tried to convince him to take this option.

Simon loved Julia his fiancée at that time and he trusted their relationship so he didn't heed his friend's advice. He told him that he can't be in a relationship with someone whom he was engaged to and then get married to someone else. He told him that it's better not to be in a relationship at all and then try that option. Simon told him that he was afraid to take the risk the second time because he have tried it the first time and it didn't work for him because he was scammed of £5,100 by someone he really trusted, living with him who promised to help him. He told him he won't take the option, he had better wait.

His friend had told him the process it involved and that he won't necessarily have to get married to the European Union lady he will be paid whom he will be introduced to. He told Simon that an immigration solicitor will have to be involved with the process and he said they have one who does the process for every applicant he had known who was granted leave to remain in the UK.

Although Simon was still under some pressure because he was scared and very careful in his daily life because he was working illegally in the UK at that time and he heard stories of how people are being rounded up by immigration officials at their place of work. Simon also heard about how people who get involved in sham weddings are often arrested. At that time he tried to talk to his fiancée to see if they could have their wedding brought forward instead of waiting for close to a year and a half, but she insisted that they should leave it at the date they had agreed on.

Simon told her his concerns at that time but she told him nothing will happen to him. Simon continued living with fear and hoped at that time that he won't be caught and sent back to Nigeria. Simon and Julia keep attending church from time to time and living happily with the kids and seeing her family members. Meanwhile at this time he had stopped getting in touch with his Uncle Tejiri because he was not responsive towards him anymore. Simon didn't know where he lived even though he has asked him several times to take him to his house. He never bothered and he didn't know where Simon lived either. He preferred seeing Simon coming to meet him at his store, so because of this he was cut off from him. He only called Simon twice to find out how he was and Simon called him several times before he finally stopped calling him. Simon tried to get his fiancée involved in work by taking up a voluntary job several times but she was very lazy to work. He tried to convince her as long as he could remember.

There was a time she went to one of the hospitals in Dartford to enquire about volunteering as a health care assistant or any available voluntary job, just to get her out of the house and prepare her for employment. She spends 90% of her time mostly online on the computer or on her phone and the house was always in a mess.

Simon tried to encourage her because he noticed she was a very lazy person. Her eldest son Michael would always spend all day on the computer playing games, eating and sleeping. He didn't go out. Her son Michael was a disabled child because he was diagnosed with Asperger's Syndrome. He had wanted to join the army. Simon always encouraged him and they did get along very well. But there was a day he insulted Simon because he told him to try and reduce the time he spends on the game console and try to find other things to do to engage himself because it will improve his personality and help in other areas of his life but he told Simon that he will slap him if he ever say such thing to him again. Since that time Simon avoided trying to tell him anything next time. If he had wanted to pass anything or say something to him after that time, he would tell his fiancée who will then speak with him instead. Simon never approached him directly after that time.

CHAPTER NINE
RELATIONSHIP BREAKDOWN

Simon and Julia's relationship as an engaged couple blossomed until he started noticing some of Julia's behaviours. Julia started getting some late night texts from people Simon didn't know and sometimes when she took a call from her phone she wouldn't want to talk in Simon's presence, she would go to a corner to talk and finish her call. Simon became worried and suspicious of her. Simon had asked her on one occasion who were the people always texting her and calling her at odd hours, she would just reply to him that they were just friends of hers. He was not satisfied with the answers she gave him because it continued even though he had felt concerned and became jealous.

So one fateful day on Sunday 26th December 2010, Julia went out with her friend Deborah for the night and Simon was with the kids at home. He was on Christmas break from work for two weeks till the New Year. When she left with her friend, Simon went online and opened Julia's Facebook because they both had the passwords to their accounts, and low and behold, Simon came across several conversations between her and one of her ex partners who was living in the North of England. When Simon checked the date of the conversation it was two months earlier at that time. So in other words the conversation started in October 2010 during the time they were engaged and went through until the day he saw it. Simon read the very first conversation between her and the guy he could remember vividly well like it just happened few minutes ago. In the conversation, the first one reads: "Hi Julia, how are you? I really miss you it's been a very long time". She replied to him saying "I am fine and doing well, I miss you too and where have you been"? He replied to her "I have been on my own for quite a time now and I just thought of you and wanted to know what's happening with you". She said "that's nice I have been lonely as usual being with the kids". He then wrote to her saying "I will be coming down to London to see my aunt and I would want us to meet". Simon read all the conversations through and when he checked the date of the conversation towards the end it was around early December 2010. Then she replied too him saying "You know I wouldn't want us to meet at my place as usual, so tell me where I can meet you". He then replied saying "I will get a hotel where you will come to meet me". Then she said "I just can't wait". He then said "I would love to make love to you once again because it's been a while, I want to taste that your wet "pussy" once more". She then said "that would be nice I just can't wait in fact you are making me horny and wet already". He then said "That's what I want to know". She then asked him when are you coming so I can come meet you at the hotel and where in London would that be? He then said "I will find a nice place or where would you prefer"?

She then said "anywhere nice and quiet". He then told her that he will book a hotel for three days between Wednesday 15th December and Friday 17th December 2010 and he told her that he would like her to spend the three nights with him. She then told him that she wouldn't be able to spend the night with him because of the kids but they can have good love making during the day for three days while the kids are at school and she wrote in the message saying "besides I won't spend the night with you because I have a friend who always visits me every weekend, so I need to stay with her. She was referring to Simon to her ex-partner as a friend and referring Simon to be a woman. She then gave him her phone number and told him to call as soon as he gets to London.

At this time Simon started shaking reading through the mails and thinking what's really going on here. He started wondering if he was reading the wrong person's mails. He went through the beginning of the mail again and read up to where he had stopped earlier, he began to ponder again. He was really confused. He checked the number she had given in the mail and checked his phone to see if it corresponds with hers or maybe she used a different number. But it was the same number. He became very mad but he still held his peace.

Then he continued reading further. Simon's fiancé Julia actually went to meet this guy in London and they had a nice time in the hotel. She wrote in a mail two days earlier before the day Simon saw the mail saying "I really miss you, it was really good love making wish I didn't have to go, I was at the train station thinking what a good and great three days I spent with you but because of the kids and my friend coming over I couldn't spend the night with you, hope you will always remember me and not just disappear again just like you left me alone and only reappearing a few weeks ago with a mail. He then replied saying "That was a great time together and I really enjoyed the sex. I will always keep in touch. I have got your number so don't worry. I will text you when I get home she said".

On Friday 17th December 2010, it was the day schools close for the Christmas break. Throughout that day Simon text Julia and tried to call her several times but her phone was switched off. When he went to her that Friday, he told her he was trying to call her and sending texts on several occasions but it says "switched off". She told Simon that the battery to her phone was dead and she was charging it.

When Simon finished reading all the messages between Julia and her ex-boyfriend, he started crying and thinking what has really gone wrong in their relationship. They had sex all the time when he was around sometimes three to four times a day she has never complained to him and he always asked her about their sex life. She always told him that no one has ever made love to her the way he used to. She told him that she has told her friend Deborah several times that he is very good in love making and he satisfies her just the way she wants. At this time Simon couldn't take it anymore and he had to call her daughter Chelsea and showed her the mails.

She was very surprised. She asked him if he is really sure it's her mother who wrote it? He told her to take a close look at the Facebook account once more who else had that account and he told her to confirm the number in the mail which she recognised as her mum's. She was dumbfounded when she saw this she was really angry and ashamed. She then told Simon to wait until her mother comes back then he should confront her with the mails and ask her to explain the meaning of everything and why she would go to meet up that guy in the hotel. She then told Simon that she knows the guy very well, his name was Benjamin. She told him that her mother was dating the guy and she introduced him to the kids but suddenly he disappeared and went to live up North of England and never communicated to her. She said her mum tried to reach him but could not and she has been living on her own not hearing from him for a very long time so she is just very surprised that they are in contact again and she didn't tell anyone. She told Simon she was really sorry about what had happened and she advised him that when he confronts her and she didn't come out with a good explanation why did that happen or beg for forgiveness then he should call off the relationship.

At this time calling off the relationship was supposed to be an ideal thing to do but because he loved her so much he didn't see that as an option. Simon made up his mind to forgive her but wanted to wait to hear why she did what she did. He waited patiently for her to come so he could confront her. But meanwhile Chelsea went to inform the eldest son Michael and he came to Simon and said he is very sorry for what had happened and he asked him if he could read the mails. Simon opened her Facebook account and he read it. Michael was very disappointment after he finished reading it and he asked Simon, what is going to be his decision. Simon told him he doesn't know but would like to speak with her when she comes back. He told the kids that he still love their mother.

Late that night Julia arrived at about 2am. Her friend had dropped her off. Simon was waiting in the sitting room patiently when she dragged herself into the house. She was very drunk, she went up the upstairs half way and sat down and started sleeping on the stairs. Simon went to check on her and saw her sleeping on the stairs he was not surprised to see her in that state but he was angry deep down. He woke her up and tried to move her to the couch to put her to sleep. But she couldn't sleep properly because she was heavily drunk. In few minutes she stood up immediately and ran upstairs to the toilet and started vomiting. She vomited for almost 20 minutes and Simon stayed with her cleaning her up.

Her son Michael was awake playing his usual video game late that night. Simon flushed the toilet several times because she vomited so many times. After some hours her eyes were beginning to clear. The first thing she said to Simon was that she was sorry for coming home drunk and promised it will never happen again. She thanked him for staying with her and helping her. He asked her if she was alright. She said "Yes I am ok now". Then he told her that there is something he would like to

discuss with her and it's very important but they should go to bed and in the morning he will explain to her.
She told Simon that she can't sleep anymore and asked what the matter was. Simon told her he can't tell her because of her state because she is just getting herself right after coming home drunk. So he suggested they go down stairs, watch TV and maybe fall asleep from there. But she insisted that he tell her because now she was troubled hearing him saying it's important and besides she has never seen such a kind of look in his face before. She kissed Simon and asked him if he was ok and placed her hands on his face. Then Simon broke it. He asked her who Benjamin was. She told Simon he was someone in her past and she has got nothing to do with him anymore.

Then she asked Simon how he came to know about him and what the matter was. Then Simon brought out his laptop opened it and went to her Facebook and showed her the conversations between her and Benjamin and how they met in a hotel, then he told her to read it and explain to him what those conversations meant. She read a bit of it and then started deleting all the messages immediately. Simon noticed her deleting it and he asked her what she was doing, she said "I am deleting it". When she finished deleting it, she then left the laptop on the floor and turned to Simon and said "it's not what you think it's just a mere flirt between I and him and nothing was really going to come out of it" then she said "I swear we never met".

Then he asked her, "Why did you delete it then if you didn't meet him because I saw the mails and I showed it to the kids." At that point she burst into tears and started crying out loud. Simon then left her in the bedroom and went downstairs to sit and think what has really gone wrong in their relationship. Her son Michael heard his mum crying and came to him and asked him why his mum was crying and asked him if they have sorted the issue. Simon told him they are still dealing with it and he told him that she has deleted the evidence and denied ever meeting Benjamin. He shook his head and went upstairs to talk to his mother.

A few minutes later he came downstairs and said his mum would like to speak to Simon. He left the sitting room and went to meet her in the bedroom. She told him that she was sorry if she has hurt him that she swears it was just a flirt and she never met Benjamin. She didn't admit even giving her phone number out.

She started undressing herself and they made love that night. She told him to trust her that she will never flirt again and saying she never knew it will hurt him. Simon asked her to put herself in his shoes how would she have reacted if he did such to her. She kept telling him after then that she was sorry and called it a mere flirt and she couldn't explain to him why she deleted those messages because that was the proof of her cheating on Simon.

After that time he became very cautious with her and watched her every move. This was when he started on another nightmare. He couldn't cope in the relationship anymore and once again he stopped taking his medication. At that time he was thinking about his future with Julia but he still loved her at that time. He thought about the effect of breaking up, what impact it would have on his mental state. He didn't want to go into hospital for the third time. Those are what he had considered.

Simon told his very close friend Ellen about his relationship she was very sorry to hear about it. She told him it was really a difficult situation he found himself in and she said she is confused and doesn't really know how to advise him at the time but she encouraged him to stay strong and stay on his medication. She told him since he still loved her he should give her a second chance and give her time. She told him that she doesn't know how she could defend herself maybe that's why she deleted the evidence and was trying to cover up. She told him that his health remains very important and he should always take care of himself. Ellen has been a very good friend to Simon though she was not physically present or lived close to him but she has been there for him all the while even now.

Simon kept going to see Julia after then but their relationship was not how it used to be anymore. He always put an eye on her and watched everything she did. She became so uncomfortable with him being around her sometimes because she was scared she might have a text or a phone call he would want to know about.

On Saturday 31st December, Deborah invited Simon and Julia to a New Year's Eve party and they travelled to another part of Kent to spend the night. It was a very dull party that night but they still had a bit of fun. That night Julia made a promise to him that she will never hurt him and promised not to flirt with any man. She told him they should stay engaged that she really wants to get married to Simon and have kids together. He told her he still loved her and would do anything to keep her. But deep within Simon didn't trust her. He found it very hard to trust her. It was just like he had got himself trapped in an unknown world. Every time he was not with her, Simon's mind would fly thinking what she was up to at that time. Life started becoming miserable for Simon.

In January 2011, Simon told his friend Ellen about his concern and that he had stopped taking his medication a few weeks earlier. He told her about his mood and fear of a relapse of his sickness. Simon told her opting out of the relationship with Julia would have an adverse effect on his health. He told her that he was still suspecting Julia. She told Simon she hoped those are not early warning signs to his sickness. Simon told her it's not an early warning sign but he was still not convinced about trusting her but his heart is still with her. She then told him that if he wants to find out if she's still continuing been unfaithful there are ways to find out. Then she told Simon that, since Simon and Julia have each other's passwords to their Facebook accounts, then whenever he is chatting to her on Facebook, he should log into her account with another web browser and then he can see which other person she was chatting with at that time. She then asked Simon that if he happened to catch her the second time cheating then he have no choice than to break up from the relationship. "BREAK UP" that's one word he was really scared to hear.

Simon followed the advice of his friend Ellen and one day while he was chatting to Julia he logged into her Facebook with another browser at the same time and behold, he got another shock of his life. Julia was chatting with another guy called "Kevin Don Matthews" that same time as he was chatting with her. In the chat, the guy was telling her that he misses chatting with her and would like them to meet. She then replied "that would be nice". The guy then asked for her number and she quickly gave it to him. Then the guy asked her when they can meet up. She then said during the week because her boyfriend comes to visit her every weekend from Friday to Sunday so during the week would be fine to meet up. Kevin then asked Julia how he can get to her house because he has never been to Gillingham before and he will be coming from London. Julia then described how he could get to her house and told him the bus number to take when he gets to Gillingham Station. As they were chatting, Kevin then asked Julia what she would want him to buy when coming. She replied that he should get a wine or any alcoholic drink.

At this time Simon's heart started beating very fast and he was confused and started thinking what a life he was living with Julia and what sort of relationship he got himself into. At this time Julia was wearing Simon's engagement ring and she was still acting this way. Simon told her that day that he was going to bed and they will chat the next day. She told Simon sweet dreams and said to him I love you always and Simon said the same. That night he couldn't sleep he was just thinking about everything. Late at night he stood up and logged into her Facebook account to check how long they have been chatting. They started chatting just the beginning of the New Year of 2011 and that time it was the middle of the month. Simon went to work that day and couldn't concentrate he was just thinking. He had wanted to confront Julia but he was thinking of a possible break up if he did. So at that time he really didn't know what to do. He told his friend Ellen about it and she told him that he should break the relationship and stay away from Julia and she told Simon also that the most important thing was his health and he should start taking his medication again.

She told him to be strong that he will get another woman who will love him and she said Julia was not a good woman. Simon couldn't break the relationship because he loved Julia so much, so didn't follow the advice of his friend instead he decided to follow his heart. That was the terrible mistake he made.

Julia and Kevin had arranged to meet up one Wednesday because Simon was following her chat with him after that day he discovered she was chatting with him. Simon decided to confront Julia indirectly by asking her a question. He asked her that as they were engaged and he started having dates with other women behind her back what would she do? She told him that she wouldn't like it because she would feel jealous.

Simon then asked her that if he was with another woman in his apartment and she phoned him while at Simon's door to ask where he was, and he told her he was at work while he was with another woman in his apartment. Then she knocked at his door and he opened it and she saw another woman with him what would she do? She just told him that she won't be angry or suspect anything but she would want to find out why the woman was with him in the first place. Then Simon knew that was a very wrong answer she had given him and not an honest one. He then asked her that if she is going to have someone else like a male in her house when no one was around will she let him know about it. She said "YES" of course she would let him know if she is going to have any male friend around the house for a date if no one was around. She asked him why he was asking her these questions, he told her he just wanted to know. Then she said he should trust her that she will never cheat on him. She said she will not make the mistake she made earlier about the flirt with the other guy named Benjamin that they never met up. She still denied it even to that day because she had deleted all the evidence. This was the week she had already arranged to meet up with Kevin.
Then Simon kept quiet and didn't say anything. Deep in his heart he was dying. He should be taking the advice of his friend but it was very difficult at that stage. He told his friend Ellen that he was going to Julia's house on that Wednesday when Kevin will be coming around and if he met him there then he will break the relationship. She advised him not to go there and told Simon; what other evidence does he need to prove that she is an unfaithful woman. She reminded him of the first incident and how she wiped off the evidence and she told him that she will do the same thing this second time. She advised him to

break the relationship for his own good because she can't be trusted. Meanwhile during this time when Simon discovered Julia was chatting with this new guy and had given him her phone number and house address, he had asked Julia if there is anything she is not satisfied with in their relationship that she should let him know.

She had told him that she really love Simon and could not live without him and wondered how life without him and the kids would be. She told Simon that she is a happier mother, that no one has ever made her happy like this in her life. Simon asked her if she was satisfied with their sex life. She said yes absolutely she is content. Then he wondered in his heart why she was still trying to meet another man and hiding it from him and then telling him to come to see her when he was not around and when her kids are away in school, it just sound suspicious to him that she was up to something but he kept his cool and decided to wait until that day when the guy was coming to meet her.

The night before the guy was supposed to meet up with Julia they chatted again while he was observing the chat and the guy told her that he can't wait till the next day. The guy told her that he bought alcoholic drink already and will be bringing it the next day. The guy told her that he will be at Gillingham Station at 10am in the morning, she said that will be fine because the kids will be away at school at that time so it's a perfect time. Then she said she goes to pick the younger daughter at school at 3pm so therefore when it's close to that time he should be off so the kids don't come and see him.

The next morning after work Simon got himself prepared to go to his fiancée's house. He had said to himself that if he met the guy there then he will call it quits with her. He got to his fiancée's house at about midday hoping to catch her with another man. He knocked on the door and her friend Deborah had come to open the door. She was very surprised to see him so was Julia. She told him what a big surprise that she wasn't expecting him but she was very happy to see him. He got puzzled he was supposed to meet another man but he found her friend with her instead. They all chatted together and had fun but in his mind he was wondering what was really going on at that time. Then Deborah left and they had sex that afternoon until close to 3pm when she went to pick up her younger daughter from school.

She was asking him why he decided to give her a surprise visit. He just told her that he missed her. They had a nice time together and he left to go back to London that day to resume his evening shift. On his way he kept wondering what had gone wrong why he didn't find the guy. That evening Simon was chatting with Julia his fiancée again and observing her chat with other men. Then she was apologising to Kevin saying that she had to cancel the meet up with him because her friend Deborah came from Dorset the night and stayed over in her house so she can't have him around when she is around and besides it was a close one had it been that he came that her boyfriend would have met him with her because he came today and gave her a surprise visit.
Meanwhile Julia had text Kevin late that night on the phone cancelling their meet up that's why Simon didn't know if not he wouldn't have gone that day and till another day when they will fix another date. She then told him as they were chatting that day that she will have to be very careful from now on because he can come in anytime to visit her so therefore he should wait and she will find a better time when they will meet up. Simon felt so bad and also very stupid to have continued in the relationship. He started stalking on his fiancée as a result which made her very uncomfortable.

Simon went to Julia's mum one day to report to her about what Julia was doing. She was not pleased to hear about it. Meanwhile all the conversations she has had with this new guy Simon copied and stored everything in his own draft messages so he can keep as evidence in case she deleted it from her Facebook. Her mother later called her and talked to her about it but she denied everything. She didn't know he had been monitoring her chat with the other guy. Her sisters came to hear what was happening between Simon and Julia and one of them was talking to her and she told her that nothing like that had happened. Towards the end of January 2011, Simon called her mother again that he had all the evidence to show to her that Julia has been unfaithful she said alright he should bring it for her to see.

After this time her mother called her and told her that Simon had got evidence to prove that she has been unfaithful. She then told her that when Simon came to show her the evidence she should have a copy of it and keep it to show her. When Simon noticed she had said this to her mother, when she was chatting to one of her sisters on Facebook, he decided to instead show the evidence to her and not show it to her mother. Then Simon went to her and told her that he had got something to show her that she has been unfaithful to him. She told Simon she would like to see it so he showed her all the conversations she has had with Kevin and told her to explain it. She told him that Kevin was forcing to talk to her and wanted them to meet that she told him that she already had a boyfriend but he kept pestering her. She said she never gave him her phone number or house address.

Then he showed her the conversation she had with him where she gave him all her contact details. Then she quickly deleted it from her Facebook and said she never did so. Then Simon told her that he still had the evidence in his own draft folder even if she had deleted it from her Facebook. Then she told Simon to delete everything from his draft folder. She said she loves him and she was sorry that she was only flirting with him. He told her that he had been monitoring her since after the first incident because she threw the trust away and now she has given him more reasons not to trust her once more. She kept apologising and in his presence she sent Kevin a text saying that he should stop texting her that her boyfriend has found out about both of them and she said in the text that she is happy with her boyfriend and wouldn't want anything to come between her and him. Kevin then text back saying "how did Simon find out and what did she tell him?" He then said in another text that "Simon has not heard from him about their plans that he would like to speak with him to reveal everything they were planning to do".

That day they made love again and he deleted the evidence from his draft folder. She promised not to repeat the same thing again and apologise to Simon but he was still not satisfied and killing himself gradually by accepting her apology and still being in the relationship. He spent the weekend there and went back to London. Meanwhile during this time (the weekend) they went to visit Julia's mum and she was very pleased to see Simon and Julia together again and she was asking how is their relationship going and they told her that they had settled it. Simon had told Julia that he will keep it secret from that day on and not tell anyone anymore about their relationship but at the same time he still doesn't trust her but he loves her and wants her to see that beyond anything. But he was making a mistake a fatal one.

On the 3rd February 2011, Simon text Julia several times and she refused to reply then he tried to call but she didn't answer his call. She had told him earlier that she was going to see her sister-in-law and she's got an important issue to discuss with her so he thought well…maybe she was busy. Then that evening he was chatting with her while he was still monitoring if she was still chatting with any other man and Simon was chatting with one of her sisters at the same time. She was asking him what happened between him and her sister so he was explaining everything that had happened to them from December 2010. She advised him to cut off the relationship with her sister if she can't be trusted. She told Simon that he should look for a more responsible woman in his life. She said she hasn't heard from her though but she is chatting with her right now and he should wait for her to chat with her.

At that time she was chatting with her sister-in-law Helen and two of her sisters, the one whom Simon was chatting with at that time. In the conversation one of her sisters was saying what is it I heard with you and Simon that you were cheating on him. She said no she was not cheating on Simon, that he had been making her unhappy about accusations and he had been watching her in everything she does that she is not free with anyone. She told her that he had made her lose all her friends. Then she said she regretted ever meeting Simon and besides he is a Paranoid Schizophrenic person and she is afraid of him. Then her sister said "YOU BETTER GET OUT OF THAT RELATIONSHIP". She said people with such illness never get well that the illness stays on for a lifetime and they are often violent people. She then asked her if Simon has had a relapse, she said she is not sure but told her that he have been living with the illness for some years now. Her sister then told her that well….she is not going to say much anymore maybe until the time when Simon relapses and poses a danger to her and the kids then she will take her advice. At that they didn't know that Simon was seeing every conversation they were making but at the same time this

was killing his soul because that was what he feared most a break up. How was he going to cope with it?
Julia then said she doesn't know how she will tell him that she was not interested in the relationship anymore that she doesn't want to hurt his feelings. Her sister-in-law Helen told her to say it to him and get the burden off her chest. She was telling her that she will find someone else and she wouldn't want to see her living a miserable life. At this time Simon was talking to Julia and asking her if anything was wrong, he was pretending that he didn't know what was going on. Then her sister who was chatting with him earlier who advised her to get out of the relationship then told him that she has just spoken to Julia and he should not worry everything will be fine.

At this time Simon felt like crying. What a hypocrite! Then Julia told him that she was not interested in him anymore and its over between them. He should have broken it a long time ago himself instead of waiting until this time and it hurts so much more than anything for her to tell him that it was over. Simon tried to convince her to chat to her and asked if he can call her on phone so they could speak but she said no she is not changing her mind. Everything he said to her at that time she was passing it to her sister-in-law on the chat while she was advising her on what to say. He felt so miserable at that time and felt the World was ending that moment. So Simon's relationship with Julia ended that day.

Then he told her that he would like to come the next day which was Friday 4th February 2011 to come and collect his belongings from her house. She told Simon she will help him pack everything and put it on the sofa in the living room, so when he comes he will just get it and leave. That night he couldn't sleep he got up at his usual 3:30am to prepare to go to work. When he got to work he told his friend about his break up with Julia who had told him earlier when he was still with Julia that he would help him arrange for someone to marry him so he could get his legal right to live in the UK. He was not very happy with Simon. He told him that he had advised him earlier to have an alternative but he have refused. He told Simon that, that very first time he caught her cheating he should have broken it long time instead of still staying with her. He said now she is bringing excuses because she wanted to do what she wants to do and it seems he stands in her way. He told Simon that he was the cause of it for giving her more chance. He then said he will help him arrange to meet his brother to find someone to get married to and pay for the service. So he helped him arrange to meet with his brother who was involved in sham marriages.

That evening he went to Julia's house after work and packed all his belongings and came back to London. He was really depressed. He started thinking about his life once more and blaming himself he should have listened to advice. Now it seems like he was on the losing side. He started having worries about his health because he couldn't sleep during the night. But Julia never stopped there she kept texting Simon asking if he was alright and that she misses him and still had feelings for him. Simon would ignore her several times and at a point in time he told her to stop contacting him and leave him alone but she would not stop she would ask if he was free so he can come online that she wants to chat with him. But he kept ignoring her and didn't say anything to her. At a point in time he got angry and replied her to stop texting him and they got into an argument on texting each other. But she never stopped texting Simon every now and then finding if he was alright.

Meanwhile Simon went to meet his friend's brother who had told him that he will help him get someone to marry him and it will cost him eight thousand pounds. He told him the procedure and everything that was involved. But he was a bit scared because he had a very bad experience of this kind in the past so he was wary about everything. Simon didn't have the eight thousand pounds at that time so he decided to take out a loan for the second time. But he was denied a loan because of his credit rating, so he was looking out to loan sharks to try and get a loan that time. But the interest rate was too high and not just that they could not offer him a loan either. Because Simon didn't want to borrow money he will find it difficult to pay back, he decided to wait and save up the money himself and then pay for the sham marriage to take place. He started saving money from that time. But Julia kept on disturbing Simon every day with text until the 9th March 2011 when she sent the last text and stopped texting Simon because he had ignored her all along.

CHAPTER TEN
THIRD RELATIONSHIP

After Simon's break up with Julia things didn't go well with him, his mental state started deteriorating gradually because of the stress he went through that time. He found it very hard to eat or sleep and he became very restless all the time. He decided to try his luck in one of the dating websites again and he joined the first one he had registered on when he met Jessica.

Simon was on the site a couple of weeks when he met another lady call Wendy. They had been chatting for a few weeks when they decided to meet. Wendy had got three kids but only two were living with her. The eldest one lived on her own. Wendy was separated from her husband some few years ago when he met her. She was 48 years old when Simon met her and he was 32 years and 4 months at the time.

Simon liked Wendy before they met right from when they were chatting. Simon travelled every two weeks to see Wendy because she lived far from London. A few weeks after they met, Wendy went through Simon's old Facebook posts and found out that he was once engaged to Julia some time ago and then she added her to her Facebook and told Simon about it. Simon was very furious about it and he asked her what she had wanted from her. Simon told her the story about him and Julia and he wouldn't want her to know anything about him. She told him that she didn't know that they once dated she just fancied having her as a friend.

Meanwhile Wendy and Julia started chatting behind Simon's and Wendy had told her that they were dating. Simon had told Wendy about his immigration status earlier and she had told him to move in with her while she speeds up her divorce. Simon had refused to move in with her because he didn't want to stay doing nothing while she feeds him and just sit at home. At that time Simon have no legal status in the UK. The job he was doing at that time paid him well to some extent so it will be wiser to continue in the job because his employer had not checked his documents to see that they had expired. After some time Simon noticed that he has made a mistake again dating someone he really didn't know very well. He discovered that Wendy was a sexaholic and wanted to be using him as a sex object every time. Simon didn't really gain anything in his relationship with her other than sex all the time. Their relationship at that time was based on sex and nothing more. Although that time his health was not stable but he didn't tell Wendy that he had a medical condition because he didn't know how she will take it and he might lose her.

During that time Simon switched off from the dating site where he had met her and he told her to do the same since they have started a relationship. But she refused she told him that her paid membership still runs on the site so she will have to wait until it expires before she would switch it off. Simon was not comfortable with it, so he tried to convince her to switch it off because it's of no point letting it run while they have started a relationship but all his effort was in vain so he kept quiet about it hoping that she will switch it off when the paid membership expires.

Since Simon was not comfortable with it he decided to set up a new profile to chat to her under a different name. And lo and behold as he was chatting with her, he asked her if she was in a relationship. She said "NO". Then he asked her what she is on the site for she told Simon that she is looking for sex. She said she gets sex though but not very often so she was looking for someone who would be satisfying her all the time. Then he told her that he will get back to her later. Then she left her number with him to call her anytime and the number she gave Simon was exactly her number. At this time he was very angry and he called her on phone and told her that the person she was chatting to a few minutes ago was him and he can see the games she was playing and he didn't trust her anymore. She started crying on the phone and told him that she was sorry and she won't do such a thing again. She begged Simon to forgive her and told him that she really loved him and doesn't want to lose him. She told him to move in with her so they can live together.

At this time he knew he had moved from a bad to a worst case scenario. Simon couldn't help it and didn't know what to do. He started thinking about his immigration status and his life at that time. Simon's life has been in mess and his health condition was not getting any better. He told his friend Ellen about all the things he was facing and she asked him if he was taking his medication he told her that he had stopped taking it a long time ago. Simon told her he couldn't sleep and eat properly and the situation of his love life is not helping matters. She advised him to cut off the relationship with Wendy and start taking his medication again. She told him that if he fall sick again the third time then he was going to lose the relationship he was trying to protect. He had thought that staying in a relationship will give him a form of security helping him to get his legal right to remain in the UK. He had thought that he wanted to look for a relationship where he can build trust and live together.
He got so lonely most of the time and had very few friends at that time most of them he didn't get to meet up with often because of their busy schedule or some of them are service users just like himself and were in and out of hospital some times more than him, so he couldn't get anybody to always spend the time with that's why he had decided to look for a partner. She told him that he

should be patient and not put himself under any unnecessary pressure. She told him that he is a faithful young man who was hard-working, a man with a good vision and someone who could take up responsibility.
She told him not to be afraid of anything that the right woman will come for him at the right time. But he was getting impatient and afraid that he might get caught one day and be deported to Nigeria.

Simon and Wendy continued to date and one day Julia sent him a message telling him that she misses him and would want them to meet to discuss. She started telling him that he should remember how they were together at the beginning when they first started a relationship. He was dumbfounded when he saw her message but he ignored it. Then after about two days she sent Simon another message asking why he had been ignoring her that he should please reply to her and that she has missed him so much. He thought about the situation and thought that, he and Julia once had a perfect relationship quite alright at the beginning!! And if she is asking for forgiveness and wants him back can't he give her a second chance? But he had thought that he was in a relationship with Wendy already, how can he go back to Julia? They had both been unfaithful, and then he started to ponder about it. Then he replied to her that he had lost trust in her a long time ago but she should give him time to think about it then he will get back to her soon. At this time he continued seeing Wendy but his trust for her has been lost for a long time. He was just in the relationship with her just watching her too see if she will still be unfaithful then he can go back to Julia.

Meanwhile Julia and Wendy had been very good friends on Facebook and they chatted all the time. Then he went to meet Wendy one weekend and she asked him if Julia sent him a message and if he ever replied to her, he told her no. but it was Wendy who had told Julia to send

Simon those messages. She said she was done with Simon and didn't know how to dispose of him so therefore they should make plans together and create a problem to set him up. Wendy then showed him the message Julia sent him and the message he sent to Julia and she told him that now who can be trusted?
At this time Simon started begging Wendy to forgive him that he was sorry for replying to Julia. He told her that he had not trusted her enough and he felt that Julia has sent him a message asking him to forgive her and she wants them to meet so he got tempted in replying her. She said she has forgiven him but she will have to put an eye on him. But at the same time Simon was angry with Julia for planning with Wendy to set him up.

Simon wrote Julia an email and told her to leave him alone and asked her what she wants from him. He told her that he was in peace with his new girlfriend why would she try to set him up? She replied that Simon was a disgraceful man and that did he ever tell Wendy that he was a Paranoid Schizophrenic person? She said who would want to be with someone with mental illness. She said Simon only needed her to get his legal right in the UK that's the reason why she changed their wedding day and moved it forward and not the reason she had given him earlier. She said he should leave Wendy alone and go and live his Schizophrenic life alone. She told him that when they were together her kids never liked him because he doesn't interact with them that he just stayed and stared at them. She said Simon got too much attached to her. Simon began to wonder because this is not true it's just an excuse for her to cover up with the things she was doing. He was very good to the kids and they were close to each other and besides what she said about him and the kids weren't true. He had thought if there has been anything like that she would have told him earlier when they were still dating.

Simon knew all these were lies. Then at this time he knew she never loved him in the first place. That day he left Wendy's place and came back to London. When he got home Wendy had sent him an email already telling him that it's over between them. Every day that passes by he would read again and again the messages Julia had sent him and ponder about it and try to think if really he was a bad person. Simon did all he had to do in his relationship with Julia and while they were together she never pointed out all this to him why then now? Julia had sent Simon all the discussions she had with Wendy through email and she mocks Simon several times thereafter.

CHAPTER ELEVEN
MY THIRD EPISODE

At this time Simon had another episode which was his third time. He started hallucinating again and became fearful of people. Simon still remembers, at this time he sent Julia a message telling her that he wanted her back and they should meet up to talk. She replied to him that she was not interested that her family won't even allow such a thing to happen. Simon wouldn't sleep at night sometimes he would take the night bus and move from one end to the other until its 3:30am when he would resume work again.

He told his friend Ellen about his health condition and she booked a flight from Rome to London just to come and spend the time with him. Ellen has been the mother around Simon and a very close friend. When Ellen was around it appeared his symptoms were reduced because she was with him always talking to him and advising him as a mother. She did all the laundry for him and cleaned his flat for him. She took him out shopping and brought after shaves for him, clothes and took good care of him. It was the first time he ever met Ellen in person. Ellen is a friendly, outspoken and outgoing person. At that time she ensured he took his medication and she was like a carer to him at that time. Ellen spent a week with Simon and they enjoyed each other's company. Two days before Ellen was to travel back to Rome, Simon received a letter from the UKBA (Home Office) telling him to report at an immigration centre in Old Street in East Central London as a regular routine check. When he read the letter he was very scared, confused and wondering how come the Home Office got his address.
He showed Ellen the letter she became very depressed and concerned about him. It was almost time, she was leaving and this bad news came, she shed tears and

wondered how come they sent him a letter from the Home Office. He had been living as an illegal immigrant for almost three years and he had changed his address two times. At that time it was a mystery how they got to know Simon's address. So he decided to seek advice from friends on what to do. What he had dreaded for many years has started hunting him the "Home Office". Simon got advice from friends who told him to write to the Home Office if he was not able to make the appointment on the day Simon was told to report and get a doctor's report to support it. On the day Ellen was leaving she left him with £30 and he saw her off to Victoria Coach Station where she took a coach to Stansted Airport. She had told Simon that she will keep calling him to know how the situation with everything was with him.

That night because he was scared to sleep in the house fearing that immigration officers might come to knock at his door he decided to sleep in the night buses and would take a bus from one end to where it terminates to another and back again. When it was morning Simon went to work and spoke with a co-worker to see if she can allow him to stay in her extra bedroom for one month until he got another apartment to rent. She asked him why he was leaving his present place he told her that the Home Office wrote him a letter to be reporting on a regular basis at a reporting centre so he was scared that when he goes to report he might be put in the plane and sent back to Nigeria.

There have been cases whereby people go to report and they are sent back to their country of birth and there have been cases whereby they could be reporting for years until maybe they will be granted leave to remain in the UK. Simon didn't know what his case would be that's why he was scared of going to report. She agreed and told Simon to move into her extra bedroom until the month ends. This was in August 2011. At that time he drafted a letter addressed to the Home Office and he went to get a report from his doctor and sent to the Home Office telling them why he missed the appointment. Simon had complained to his doctor that he have constipation which have prevented him from travelling to the reporting centre at that time and will report as soon as the condition relieves him.

Simon started living with Lorraine at that time who was his co-worker. She was a single parent with three kids. They lived happily together with the kids at that time he felt at home because the kids were nice to him so was Lorraine and they took him as a family member but at this time he had already relapsed the third time but he was just coping with the situation. Because he was not on the streets and he lived with people who cared for him the symptoms at that time were reduced. Although he still continued to see his carer at the early intervention service. He told his friend Ellen about his new home and she was very happy and encouraged him to keep taking his medication. He lived with Lorraine for up to a month as he said he would and her boyfriend spoke on her behalf that she doesn't want him to go that he should continue staying in her house but he should be paying £220 every month for the room. So he agreed and he continued staying there.

In early October 2011, Simon went to another dating site and met a lady call Barbara, she was a Canadian and they are friends up till today but he didn't stay long on the site because he switched off from it due to his paranoia. Barbara is Simon's godmother she is just like Ellen. She's got a son Simon's age and she advises him on personal issues and knows him very well. They talk almost every day. But meanwhile Simon met another girl name Rachel she was an American. They got chatting and agreed to meet up. She was planning to come visit him in the UK in 2012. Because he was so desperate at this time looking for all opportunity to get a legal status and wanted to run away from the UK, Simon and Rachel agreed to get married when she visits him in the UK and then when she goes back to America she can then apply for him as a spouse to come join her in America.

Simon was so scared that something might happen to him in the UK since the Home Office are now involved in his case. During this period he had already relapsed but he didn't know because he could still do everyday tasks but the way he thinks and perceives things was different from a normal human being. Rachel lived with her parents who live with their parents at that time in Tennessee in the USA. But because she was looking for a job and wanted to travel to North Dakota where she would find a job she needed money to make the journey and her parents could not afford to get her the money.
So Simon decided to send her $400 cash through DHL to assist her in getting to North Dakota. She received the money and thanked him and her mother was very happy and thanked him too. She got to North Dakota and stayed with a friend's mother. She sent Simon a present in the post which was a Christian DVD movie, a T-Shirt, Men's Devotional Bible and a portrait of her photo. But two days after she got to North Dakota she sent Simon a message that she was not interested anymore in a relationship with him and she was very sorry. Her mother was very concerned because she saw the status change on her daughters Facebook account from being in a relationship to single and she wrote Simon to ask what had happened between him and her daughter Rachel. Simon explained everything to her how they met and how they plan to get married when she visits him in the UK the following year. She was not happy and promised to get back to him.

The day the present came to be delivered Simon wasn't at home so he was left with a note for a missed delivery which asked him to come collect it at the depot with an ID. But he felt it was of no point to go collect it and thought if it stays for more than 20 days it will be shipped back to the sender. Meanwhile before this time Simon's employer have started checking files of all the employees and ordering those whose documents have expired or about to be expire to bring a renewed documents from the Home Office. At that time Simon contacted one of his friends he knew when he was working at the club years back to help him produce a doctored document so he could take it to his employer so he can continue working. She introduced him to a man who helped people with fake documents in Southeast London and he told Simon it will cost him £400 to get a fake document. Simon paid him £400 to help him get a document so he could take to his employer and that was the last time he ever saw him. The man ran away with his money. He was in the same situation with Simon, having no legal right to live in the UK but he does fake documents for other illegal immigrant to work in the UK. That is how he survives.
It was a very bad time for Simon that period. It just seemed that everything he tried to do at that time was failing. This causes more and more stress for him and was affecting his thinking.

So with the stress and fear of the Home Office getting him, he started hallucinating. He was thinking that the Queen of England can give him a passport. He started seeing himself as a diplomat of the UK. He started hearing voices again and thinking he had a special power. He went to see his carer at the early intervention service and told her that he wants to write to the Queen and how should he address it. He sent his new passport which he just got from the Nigeria High Commission at that time with a letter to Balmoral Castle in

Aberdeenshire asking for the Queen to accept him as a royal guard. Simon became confused and frustrated. This was how his nightmare began for the third time. During this time it was like commentaries are been run through his thought. He read the newspapers and every statement he read was like it talks about him. He couldn't cope with his thoughts he struggled to come to terms with reality.

Simon's third episode was very similar to his second. It was a terrible and fearful experience he had at this time. He was trying to hide his thoughts from himself because at this time it was like the voices became more and more persistent in speaking to him and finding out what he was thinking. During this time he used to think that anything he had in his thoughts or was thinking about was been taken to the Home Office by the voices. Also he started to fear that his exes knew his whereabouts and could read his mind from wherever they are. He could not find a way of getting out of his situation because during this period he was vulnerable and sick.
One night when the voices were speaking to him, he heard another gentle voice telling him to call the ambulance to take him to hospital. But another voice told him that he should not call the ambulance and he should remember the incident in the library when he assaulted a young lady and the police came around. He also heard the voices telling him that he should remember his second episode where police got involved so calling an ambulance is not an option. He became so confused and started thinking about his immigration status, thinking he might get into trouble if he called the ambulance. The voices in his head at that time began to talk between each other while he listened. This was a terrible and horrible experience. Simon stood up walked around the house to see if the voices will die out but it became persistent. He tried to sleep but couldn't. He had not had

his medication before this time for a long time so he became restless.

The voices at that time were talking in his head to each other, one was saying that he was weak and he will die and saying he had a very big problem with the Home Office and he had nowhere to run to. The other was saying that he should remain calm and things will be sorted. He was so helpless and didn't know how to keep the voices silent in his head. He got angry at a time and he screamed to himself shouting "ENOUGH" then he quickly picked up the phone and dialled 999. An operator picked up the call and asked who does he want the police or an ambulance. He quickly said ambulance and he was connected to an ambulance service. A lady picked the call and asked what the problem was. He told her that he hears voices in his head and it's been persistent for a while now and he was very confused so he needed a doctor to help him with the voices. She took his name, date of birth and address. She asked him if he have a carer and he replied "YES". She asked him what medication he was on and when was the last time he took it. Simon told her it's been a long time ago. She then said the hospital is a noisy place to be and it's full that he should stay at home and remain calm and said he should try to go to bed and if the voices come back to his head again then he should phone back again then the ambulance will come and take him to the hospital.
At this time Simon felt relieved and the voices died down a bit but they were still speaking to him because he could hear them faintly saying if he goes to the hospital he will be injected with the wrong medication and he will die. The voice started telling him that he was close to his death. Simon became scared and dared not to call the ambulance for the second time because he believed the voices. That night he couldn't sleep, he had just a few hours' sleep after the torment and at 3:30am his landlady woke him up so they could go to work. He shouted at

her that he was already at work. At that time, he had thought that listening to the voices was his job so he need not go to work anymore. She became scared of him because he had never been in such a mood before. So she left him alone and went to work.

That morning he booked an appointment to see his doctor (GP). Simon told him that he heard voices and it was so strong the previous night that he had to scream to keep them quiet. He then gave Simon a prescription and told him to book an appointment to see his Psychiatry Doctor. He told Simon he shouldn't have stopped taking his medication and he said he was having a relapse. But Simon never thought so he just thought at that time that he was going through stress and he will get over it. So he left his doctor and went back home to rest. While he was on his way he received a phone call from his employer telling him to report at their office and he should not go back to work the next day and when he is coming to see them, he should bring his renewed Home Office documents if he had them.

Then he heard the voices again telling him that he should not go that the Home Office are waiting to get him at his employer's office. He became so scared and worried. He had thought that the Home Office has been contacted by his employer and will be there when he report. Then he began to ponder about it and he made up his mind to go despite been scared. He had thought that he can't afford to lose his job because that will make him homeless again because he will have no money to pay for his rent and feed himself. At that time he didn't know that he had already relapsed from his illness.

So Simon went to his employer the next day and he was asked to produce his passport and a valid visa but he told them that he didn't have any. He told them that the Queen is going to issue him a UK passport so he was waiting for it. They seemed confused and asked him how come the Queen will give him a passport. He told them that he was a UK citizen that he is waiting for it to be approved and it's only the Queen that can solve his immigration problem. Then they asked him how he came to the UK and he told them that he came initially as a student and his visa ran out in December 2008. So he had been trying to renew it since then. They asked him why he haven't renewed his visa after it had expired a long time ago, and they told him that they were going through each employee's file and updating it because the Home Office officials had started coming to do routine checks on the company. They said they noticed that Simon's visa had expired three years earlier and they didn't want to fall victim because the Home Office could fine them for employing an illegal immigrant. They told Simon that though he is very punctual to work and he is a very hard working employee they could not take the risk of employing him so therefore they are terminating his appointment and he can come back to work after he had renewed his visa with the Home Office. They told him they will pretend they don't know where he lives and will not report him to the Home Office.

So Simon left his employer's office that day thinking what will be the next step for him. He was really down and thinking how he will survive without a job. He knew he was in with another big trouble in front of him. He started thinking about his homelessness when he just came into the UK. He decided to go see his Psychiatry Doctor as advised by his doctor (GP). He booked an appointment and luckily for him the doctor was around that same day. So on that day he was made to wait for few minutes at the Early Intervention Service to see his care worker. Simon was later invited into a room and seated in the room was the Psychiatry Doctor, his care coordinator and four other mental health professionals. Simon's

Psychiatry Doctor began to ask him some questions. He asked Simon when the last time he took his medication. Simon told him a long time ago that he can't remember. He asked him to explain why he came the other day and asked one of the carers on how to address a letter to the Queen of England. He told him that his immigration problem is the main problem to his mental health and if that is solved he will be free from worries and he will live a normal life like every individual. Simon told him that he had been struggling with mental health issues over the years and he can't go back to Nigeria because it will be worse there and he will die like his elder brother who died in 2003 with the same illness.

Therefore he believes the Queen will give him a British passport and make him a citizen. He asked Simon why did he believe that the Queen alone that can give him a British passport. Simon told him that it's only the Queen that will listen to him that she is kind and of pure spirit. He told him that the Prime Minister is against him and doesn't want him to succeed. He told him that he is suspicious of everyone except the Queen, that's why she is the only one to help him become a citizen of the UK. He then asked Simon if he hears voices recently. He told him "YES" I do. Then he told him to tell him what the voices have been saying to him. He told him that the night before he heard different voices talking to him that he will die and he has no legal right to be in the UK, then he heard another voice saying that he will not die but should remain calm. Then at a point he shouted to the voices verbally to keep them quiet then he called the ambulance to take him to hospital. He asked Simon that why does he want to go to hospital? Simon told him that hospital is the place where you go to and leave the voices and return home without hearing them, that's why he had thought of going to the hospital.

He then asked Simon that does he think anything is wrong with him. Simon told him that "NO" he was alright he just think he needed a rest and he was going through stress. He then asked Simon how his appetite was. Simon told him that he had not been eating well because of the stress and the voices he heard scared him a lot. Simon told him that he was really worried about his condition because he suspected everyone since they are trying to kill him and planning against him. He then asked Simon does he think that he is planning against him. Simon told him that he was not too sure about that but he was watching him. He then said ok, at this time he said he should give them a break to decide what to do with him and they will come back to him in few minutes.
Simon was left alone in the room with only one of the mental health professional. In the room she told him that he should be calm and everything will be fine with him. She kept assuring Simon and smiling at him each time. After a few minutes his Psychiatry Doctor came in with his care coordinator while the other four mental health workers didn't return and they sat down. He then asked Simon how he felt. Simon told him that he was feeling not too different but a bit relaxed but just thinking what will happen from then. He then said Ok.

He told Simon that he will give him two options to choose from. He told Simon that they will either get him to the crisis team, whom he will be going to see every day and they will ensure that he takes his medication every day and they will be monitoring his progress or he can choose to go into hospital. Simon had thought at that time that he didn't want to go to the crisis team but had no reason to explain to himself why.

On the other hand he had thought that it was a plan by his Psychiatry Doctor, his care coordinator and the other four mental health professionals who left the room earlier, that they knew he won't like to go to the crisis team and won't take the hospital option either. So they have come up with difficult options to choose from where they will force him to go to hospital and then inject him with a medication that will kill him, "NO WAY". Then Simon replied that what if he refuses to take either of the two options what will happen? Then his Psychiatry Doctor told him that they will have no option than to force him into hospital. Then the voices started speaking to him again telling him that he should find a way of escape that he was going to be killed in the hospital that it's a plan.

Simon started been scared and worried. His Psychiatrist noticed this and he assured him that nothing will happen to him and asked why he was been scared to go to the crisis team or the hospital. Simon told him that he doesn't trust anyone anymore. He said he will get killed in the hospital. He told Simon that he won't be killed that he will get treatment and get well. He assured him that nothing bad will happen to him that he will be in safe hands. He told Simon that his care coordinator will be coming to check on him during ward round and he will be seeing him as well during the ward round. As he tries to convince Simon, the voices spoke to him at the same time telling him he was doomed. Before he knew it, he was taken to an ambulance waiting outside the building and he was driven to St Pancras Mental Health Hospital in King's Cross in North London in the borough of Camden. This was in November 2011. So Simon was admitted in hospital for the third time for relapse of his Schizophrenic episode.

In the hospital Simon was taken to a ward on the ground floor and showed his room. One of the staff nurses on duty showed him the toilet and shower room in his room and how to use it and told him if he need any help he should let any of the nurses on duty know. He then gave Simon a form and told him he should fill it if he felt that

he was brought into the hospital without an illness in other words if he wants to appeal against his section under the mental health act. He also gave him a list of mental health solicitors he can contact and told him he had only two weeks to make the appeal if not he will continue to remain in hospital under the section he was under until he gets well or discharged from the hospital.
At this time Simon's landlady learnt he was in a Psychiatry hospital and he had lost his job so she called him on the phone to come and collect his belongings from her house. The next day was ward round and the Psychiatrist came to the ward. He saw some patients and Simon was told that he will be seeing him as well. During Simon's first day in hospital, he was restless because he couldn't sleep for the first few hours he was thinking that he was going to die, so he roamed the corridors of the ward watching and trying to see what other patients and nurses were doing. He was so paranoid at this time and suspicious of everyone.

He was able to sleep at night after he had taken his medication, but when he was about to sleep he locked himself in his room because he was scared that the nurses might come in to kill him.

After waiting for some time Simon was told to come into the consulting room to see the Psychiatrist. In the room was seated his Care Coordinator, Psychiatrist, one of the staff nurses on duty and two student nurses. Simon's Psychiatrist asked him why he kept roaming the corridor of the ward when he first came into the hospital. Simon told him that he wanted to see what the nurses are up to because he heard a voice telling him that they are preparing a medicine to inject him so he will die. He told him that no one will kill him that he was safe in the hospital. He then asked him why he didn't think that the voices he hears are not true. He said the voices have been speaking to him for a very long time that things will happen but did not happen then why did he keep worrying over them. Simon told him that it might happen one day. Then he said “NO” it won’t happen.

He asked Simon if he still heard voices and if he slept well the previous night. Simon told him yes he had slept well and that he still hears the voices that’s why he has been on his toes watching everyone in the ward. He asked him if he still thinks that the Queen will give him a UK passport. He told him “YES” he still had that strong feeling that the Queen will give him a passport. He then asked Simon that if the Queen will give him a UK passport, how she will do that. Simon told him that he will have to apply through the Home Office to the Queen. Then Simon told him that the Queen is going to take over the Home Office and she will have the right to decide who she will grant a passport. He asked Simon if he have passed the Life in the UK test. Simon told him that he doesn’t need to write it that it will be a waiver for him by the Queen. He then said Ok. He then told Simon that they will not have a long discussion but he will be transferring him to another ward because that ward is not the ward for him. He told Simon that he will be in care of another Psychiatrist but although his Care Coordinator will be coming to see him on every ward round. Then he told Simon to go back to his room.

Simon left and went back to his room and stayed for a while then one of the staff nurses on duty called him to speak to his Care Coordinator afterwards. Simon spoke with her and she told him that he should not worry and he will be fine that he was in the right place. She told Simon she will be seeing him at the next ward round when he would have been transferred to another ward. She told him he should feel free with the staff nurses that they are there to help him. So she left. Simon was transferred to another ward on the top floor. He was transferred there two days after he saw his Psychiatrist.

Simon was showed his room and the staffs were very friendly and kind.

Simon continued receiving treatment in the hospital and the voices were beginning to reduce just like magic. It was the effect of the medication. He felt very happy while in the hospital. All the suspicion of hospital staff wanting to kill him lessened and he could relate well with the staff and other patients. At one of the ward rounds the Psychiatrist of the ward told him that he was doing very well and he will be discharged soon but they have nowhere to discharge him to because he can't go back to his former place where he had lived since he had gone to move his belongings with a staff nurse from his landlady's house to the hospital.

She advised him to seek legal help to sort out his immigration status because they will have to inform the Home Office that he was in the hospital. This was another issue Simon knew he have to deal with again with his mental health; it has always been the issue of his mental health and his immigration status. At this time he was given two hours unescorted leave out of the hospital to go look for an immigration solicitor to make a fresh application to the Home Office. Simon was given a list of immigration solicitors by one of the staff nurses in the ward and he chose from the list an immigration solicitor. He called the office and booked an appointment to go and see the solicitor. Simon used the two hours unescorted leave he had, which was given to him by his psychiatrist to go and see the solicitor.

On arrival at the solicitor's office, he was made to sit down for a while by the receptionist while she went in to tell the solicitor a client was waiting. After a few minutes Simon was called in by the solicitor and asked about his immigration problem. He explained to the solicitor how he came to the UK in September 2007, how he had been living in the UK, his mental health problems, how he have been refused a visa to continue to stay in the UK several times and where he was presently.

The solicitor told him that the only way he could get his right to remain in the UK was only by applying for a discretionary leave to remain in the UK. He advised Simon that based on what he had said so far concerning his story; it is not guaranteed that it will be granted. So therefore Simon didn't qualify for legal aid. Simon had been expecting to make a fresh application to the Home Office on legal aid at that time. The solicitor told him that he will be charged a Home Office fee and solicitors fee if he was interested in going ahead with the application. The solicitor asked him if he was interested in making the application. He said "YES" but he had no money. She then suggested to him to go look for friends, family members or relatives who can support him with the fee. At that time he knew no family member or even friends who could help him with money to make an application at the same time it is not guaranteed if he will be granted leave to remain in the UK.

So Simon decided to look for another solicitor. He went back to the hospital and called another solicitor from the list provided to him. He booked an appointment to see another solicitor the next day.

Simon went to see another solicitor and told him his situation and how he would like to apply for leave to remain in the UK. The solicitor told him the same thing the first solicitor had said. He said they can't help him with legal aid because his case is not strong enough or worthy to be funded by legal aid, but if he wants to make an application then he will have to pay towards it. Simon left the solicitor and went back to the hospital. At this time he was panicking and thinking how his situation will get solved. He was under enormous pressure as well because the Home Office had already known that he was in hospital. On the ward round that follows, he told his Psychiatrist that he will kill himself if the Home Office tries to come and take him out of the hospital to the detention centre. He told her that he cannot go back to Nigeria and he wanted to remain in the UK. Simon told her he needed time to look for another solicitor who will help him in his case.

Simon's Psychiatrist then told him that she will have to leave him on section under the mental health act because he was feeling suicidal. Simon's psychiatrist had wanted to lift him off section earlier since he was doing well but changed her mind when he told her that. Simon was given more time by his psychiatrist to go look for another solicitor but meanwhile he called the Home Office and told them that he received their letter they sent him since August four months earlier and he was now admitted in hospital but would like to report to an immigration officer. They told him that he should not bother he should wait until he leaves hospital and then let them know his new address and then he can report then.

Simon got very scared with that so he planned to quickly get another solicitor. Simon went through the list again and found another solicitor. Simon booked an appointment to go to see the third solicitor. At his appointment he explained to him his situation what he had already told the first two solicitors. Then he told Simon that though his case stands at a 50 50 success rate, if the application is made to the Home Office based on what he had told him so far. But nevertheless he will help him make the application and he would need a Psychiatry report from his Psychiatrist to envisage the effect of his removal from the UK would have on his mental health and also he told him that he will have to do findings in other words research on mental health services in Nigeria. He gave Simon his office card and told him to call him anytime if he had a problem. He told Simon that he should not get in contact with the Home Office and if they get in contact with him then he should tell them to speak to him. He told Simon that he will have to apply for an asylum and told him the details of the asylum process. This period was just a few days to Christmas in 2011. He told him that he will have to apply for asylum in the New Year and he assessed his financial status and told him that he qualifies for a legal aid.

He asked Simon for his Psychiatrist and his care coordinator's contact details so he can start all the paper work. Simon was very happy and it just felt like a burden has been taken off his shoulder. He went back to the hospital with a smile in his face. He informed his psychiatrist and the staff nurse that his application will be made in the New Year and they were pleased to hear that.

A few days after, Simon received a letter from his immigration solicitor advising him what to do and explaining the terms and condition as a client of the firm. Simon spent the Christmas of 2011 and New Year 2012 in hospital. It was a lovely day that day because each patient received presents from the hospital and there were lots to eat.

In January 2012, the no recourse to public funds team provided Simon with a temporary accommodation in the borough of Haringey with weekly subsistence of £35. So he was officially discharged from hospital in mid-January 2012.

CHAPTER TWELVE
MY BREAKTHROUGH

But before this time Simon had begun his asylum application earlier in January 2012 and he was scheduled to come to the Home Office in Lunar House in Croydon in two months after for a screening interview. On the day of his screening interview it was a weekend and he went to the Home Office and he spent the whole day there. He was screened and asked some basic questions about why he was claiming asylum, how he came to the UK and some other questions. At the end of the day he was told to report the next Tuesday at the reporting centre in Old Street in East central London to know when he will have his main interview.

So on the Tuesday, Simon was at the reporting centre and he was marked in the register and told to come back the following Monday for his main interview and have every supporting documents ready to submit on that day. During this period he continued taking his medication and didn't stop for one day and he still continued to see his care coordinator but he was very anxious as to what the outcome of his application would be. He started praying and attending a local church and making sacrifices to GOD.

On the day of his asylum interview, he had collected the psychiatry report and his solicitor's report and his own statement why he wants to remain in the UK and background information about mental health services in Nigeria. On that day he was interviewed by a lady called Margaret Sills. The interview took six hours with a thirty minute break. They started from 9am till noon and then had 30mins break and then started again at 12:30pm till 3:30pm. During the interview, he was asked about 350 questions. The interview was recorded on a tape and at the same time as he was answering the questions, the interviewer was writing. He was very happy with his interview because right from that moment he knew he did very well and was just waiting for the outcome.

At the end of March 2012, Simon's immigration solicitor called him and congratulated him and said his asylum application was successful so therefore he has been granted a Refugee status in the UK. He told him that he was now a legal resident in the UK and he could now work or study and live in the UK with no barrier or restrictions. Simon was so happy and speechless at that moment. He asked him if he would want anyone to know about it, he told him yes he wanted him to let his care coordinator know about it and his psychiatrist. So his immigration solicitor told them. A few minutes later his care coordinator called him to congratulate him. This was all Simon had ever wanted all along just a legal status in the UK and he got it at last after so many years of living as an illegal immigrant in the UK, it came at last. He called his family members and told them about it. Everyone was overjoyed. He has been living freely right from that moment.

Simon moved out of England in May 2012 and came to Scotland. He has been a good Christian now and rededicated his life to GOD and he attends a local Church where he lives. Now he is free from all immigration worries and he has no cause to stop taking his medication. His care has been transferred to Scotland and he now has a Community Psychiatry Nurse and a Psychiatrist whom he sees from time to time. He is now in the best mood he has ever been in because the barrier has been broken. Scotland is where he wants to live and start a new life for himself. Scotland is now his home he is very proud to be in Scotland and he sees himself as being Scottish and no one can take that from him. He now has an unconditional offer of admission to study for his Master's degree in one of the Scottish Universities in September and he has plans to go further to study for his PhD and work in research in Scotland thereafter.

SUMMARY

Thanks for taking the time to read Simon's Biography, he hopes you have enjoyed it so far? Simon grew up in a family where there was no peace with just one parent taking care of seven children. It was not an easy thing for his mother to bear. He grew up never having the love of his father; he left them when they most needed him. As you can see from the book, broken homes can lead to mental health and broken relationship as well as in Simon's case, there have been reported cases of genetic factors involved too recently. Simon felt isolated most times because he was away from his country of birth far from family and friends. He found himself in an environment where the culture was much more different from where he grew up.

Mental health (Schizophrenia) can be treated, prevented and individuals with mental health problems should never be isolated in the society. They have rights like every other person living on the face of the earth. There should be more awareness about mental health in the society. Simon also want to encourage everyone who has read this book to always accept their past without regrets, handle the present with confidence and face the future without fear. Living with mental health goes beyond just diagnosis.

At one point in time Simon has depended so much and put trust in humans and got failed. Everyone should put their trust in GOD who is the author and finisher of our faith.

Simon has decided to write this book to tell people his story and encourage people who are having mental health difficulties to remain strong. No one should think of ending his or her life because of years of treatment or suffering with mental health issues. There is always a light at the end of the tunnel. Simon has now reconciled with his elder brother and sister and they are living like family once more.

Simon wants to thank all his carers for helping him throughout the years. This is his story put together in a book call **Made in Scotland**: The Biography of the Life and Events of a Paranoid Schizophrenic Patient, because he wrote this book when he moved to Scotland and thanks for reading his story.

Finally he wants to give GOD the Glory and praise for helping him through this book.

Lightning Source UK Ltd.
Milton Keynes UK
UKOW05f2350160813

215487UK00001B/6/P